D0856043

GARDNER-WEBB COLLEGE LIBRARY
P. O. Box 836
Boiling Springs, N.C. 28017

'LUDES

A
Ballad
of
the Drug
and
the Dream

BENJAMIN STEIN

'LUDES

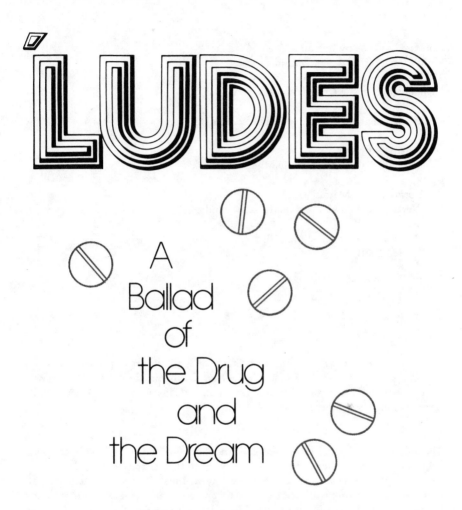

A
Ballad
of
the Drug
and
the Dream

GARDNER-WEBB COLLEGE LIBRARY
P. O. Box 836
Boiling Springs, N.C. 28017

ST. MARTIN'S/MAREK   NEW YORK

HV
5825
.S73
1982

Copyright © 1982 by Benjamin Stein
For information, write: St. Martin's Press,
175 Fifth Avenue, New York, N.Y. 10010
Manufactured in the United States of America

Library of Congress Cataloging in Publication Data

Stein, Benjamin, 1944-
  'Ludes, a ballad of the drug and the dream.

  "A St. Martin's/Marek book."
  1. Narcotic addicts—United States—Case studies.
I. Title.
HV5825.S73   363.2'93'0922 [B]   81-23192
ISBN 0-312-50012-2   AACR2

Design by Kingsley Parker

10 9 8 7 6 5 4 3 2 1

First Edition

The lines from "Voyages" I by Hart Crane on pg. 176 are reprinted from *The Complete Poems and Selected Letters and Prose of Hart Crane*, edited by Brom Weber, with the permission of Liveright Publishing Corporation; Copyright 1933 © 1958, 1966 by Liveright Publishing Corporation.

The following story is based on real-life experiences. While everything in the book is intended by the author to be true as a whole, no representation is made that any particular incident occurred exactly as portrayed. Most of the characters are patterned on one or more real people; a few are archetypical. However, no representation is made or intended that the real-life counterpart of any character did or said all of the things done or said by that character in the book. Moreover, the events described are based on actual happenings, though some actions that are attributed to one character actually involved someone other than that character's real-life counterpart.

For Colonel Dale Denman, Jr., U.S. Army, Retired,
and Norma Jean Denman.

PREFATORY NOTE:

In the writing of this story, I am indebted mostly to John H. Mankiewicz for his literary contributions. The beauteous one, Alexandra Denman, encouraged me to continue to write this book when I wanted to stop because it was too sad to relive it all. Stan Newman, Lois Wallace, Michael Chimich, and especially Dick Marek made it all seem worthwhile. Sally Richardson worked to make further work possible. She succeeded, which is rare, and I thank her.

BECALMED

Lenny Brown never leaves his room by day. He lies in his unmade bed with a bowl of Doritos next to him, on the floor. To his left, on the mattress, is an ashtray filled with smoldering cigarette butts. Above his head, to his right, the dirty white wall is marked with brown streaks from striking kitchen matches against it. On the faithful, flickering Panasonic at the foot of the bed, a fat woman wonders whether she should bet that more than fifty percent of wives thought their husbands were good lovers. A month's worth of L. A. Times are scattered across the floor. A travel poster is Scotch-taped to the wall, advertising a windmill and, by extension, the scenic beauties of Aix-en-Provence. The poster belongs to the previous tenant.

Outside, it is hot and sunny, with a pleasant onshore breeze. The boardwalk, which in Los Angeles is made of concrete, is only a block from Lenny's window. There are young girls in tight cutoffs roller-disco dancing to the music of Sony Walkmans. A young black street musician plays music to a crowd from a guitar; amplifier, batteries, and speakers all strapped to his back. He is on a skateboard. At sea, there are dozens of sailboats with brightly colored sails.

This is inside. It is still, hot, and smoky. The sliding glass windows are shut. Fifth-hand blackout drapes are pulled. The air conditioner is turned on, but it is not working properly, only poorly filtering and cooling the air from outside. The only light comes from the television, where the fat woman, who has just lost $200 betting that most wives thought their husbands were not good lovers, is about to bet again. The host offers her another wager and the fat woman starts hopping up and down. She looks like a bottle-blond rabbit in a turquoise polyester jump suit.

"I just wonder," Lenny says in a voice that sounds older than his thirty-three years, "I just wonder if you know how hard it is for most people to tell the difference between a bootleg Quaalude and a real one from Lemmon. Do you know how to do it?"

"I really don't," I say. The walls of Lenny's apartment are made of cardboard, and I can faintly hear a "Save the Whales" rally coming together on the boardwalk.

"It's simple if you know the trick," he says. "You just line up the pills on a glass-topped table." I notice that he has a glass-topped table in his one-room apartment. The table and the television are the only pieces of furniture that look as if they have not spent one hundred years on Devil's Island. "So you line up the 'ludes," he says, "and you make sure the 'Lemmon' sign, on each pill, is facing the same way. You've got to have at least ten of them for this to work. Then you look *under* the table, up through the glass, and look at the little lines that cut the pills in half." Lenny strikes a match on the wall and lights a Viceroy.

"Are you with me so far?" he asks.

His cocker spaniel, Daisy, cocks her head as if he is talking to her.

"I'm with you."

Lenny takes such a deep drag on his cigarette that in one puff he turns a third of the butt to ash. He continues. "Say you look at those little lines and they're going every which way. Remember, the trademarks on top are all lined up. But the lines on the other side *don't* line up. What would you think? Real or bootleg?"

"I don't know."

"You'd think they were fake, right? I mean, they're all different. If they all lined up, they'd be straight from the factory." Lenny puts out his cigarette. The ashtray overflows. Some old, burned filter tips fall on a dirty blue-and-white-pinstriped fitted bottom sheet. Lenny, with his left hand, absentmindedly flicks the butts back into the ashtray. The ashes remain on the sheet. He rubs them in with the palm of his hand as he talks.

"If the lines go every which way," he says, "you'd think that someone made them at home, right?"

"Yes," I say. "That's what I'd think."

"Yeah," Lenny says, "but then you'd be wrong. You see, Lemmon stamps the pills in groups of five, then they do another five, then another. Of course," he adds, "they've got a whole bunch of machines working at once. But the pills come out all screwed up, lines going everywhere. The guy who makes them in his basement in Gardena, well, he's only got one machine. So the pills all come out the same way. You'd be amazed," he says. "It's really almost unbelievable."

"What's unbelievable?" I ask.

"It's unbelievable how many people don't know how to tell the difference between a bootleg Quaalude and a real one. That's really important these days," he says.

These days keeps going through my mind while Lenny goes back to "Card Sharks" or "The $20,000 Pyramid" or "The Joker's Wild." *These days* Lenny Brown cannot get out of bed for most of the day. *These days* Lenny Brown lives in an apartment where the dirt is thick enough to write your name on; where roaches crawl along dishes with total impunity; where the only food in the refrigerator is half-full cans of Diet Pepsi, ancient scraps of lettuce long turned brown, and a jar of French's mustard with a pushdown spout—another relic of the prior tenant. *These days* Lenny Brown has just borrowed $200 from the only person who will lend him money any longer, the only person whom he will ever ask for money, basically the only friend he has. Lenny says he will pay me back soon somehow. I tell him there is no hurry, but he insists that he always pays his bills. He "may start" dealing 'ludes, in which case he will soon make so much money that he will be able to buy the building if he feels like it. He has not yet decided to start dealing, but he *probably* will. *These days.* Lenny Brown no longer has the house with the million-dollar view in the Hollywood Hills or the tobacco-brown Mercedes or the rented cottage in the Malibu Colony. *These days.*

Lenny Brown has the money I have just given him, and he is desperate. He is out of Quaaludes. That is what the $200 is for. I do not know how many 'ludes $200 will buy, but I do know that Lenny's hands are shaking.

These days the shakes keep Lenny in bed until he has had a few 'ludes so that he will not feel dizzy. The shakes make Lenny need Diet Pepsi, for reasons I know well. The shakes have forced Lenny to drink his soda through a straw. When I come to visit, which is not very often, he usually keeps his hands under the covers, except when he is smoking his Viceroys, as he is now, while he waits.

Waiting for pills is a major part of Lenny Brown's life. He needs between twelve and fifteen Quaaludes every day, and Quaaludes, according to Lenny, are not that easy to get. *These days.* "You've got to cover yourself," Lenny says. "I know five or six guys who can get them from time to time. Some can get them more than others. One guy has them practically all the time, but they're hardly ever the real thing."

Lenny reaches for the phone and dials a number he knows by heart. He lets it ring. I can hear the phone from where I am sitting, and we both sit in silence while the phone rings about thirty times. Finally, Lenny hangs up. "Great," he says, with a smile. "He's not home. That means he's on his way."

It is now early morning, and the television has flickered from game shows to news to reruns of "I Love Lucy" to "M.A.S.H." The other people in Lenny's apartment building are coming home from work, at least the ones who work. There is a thud against Lenny's door and I look over. It wasn't a knock.

Lenny sees me looking and shakes his head. "It's those kids down the hall," he says. "They're always throwing that damn Frisbee in the hallway." The kids' footsteps and laughter disappear, and Lenny and I watch "M.A.S.H." In Lenny's apartment the laugh track on "M.A.S.H" seems unusually loud.

"I've seen that one before," says Lenny. "I really like 'M.A.S.H.' It's an incredibly well-produced show. I think someday down the road, I might get into TV production. There's a lot of money in it." Lenny picks up the phone and dials the number. He hangs up quickly this time. "It's busy," he says, "but not the kind of busy signal you get when people are talking. It's a faster tone. That means someone else is calling in. He'll be here any minute," Lenny says. "This guy's never late."

"What time was he supposed to be here?" I ask.

There is a knock on the door. I glance over at the door. When I turn around to look at Lenny, I gasp. He has taken his Python pistol from under his covers and is pointing it at the door. It is visibly trembling in his hand.

"What the hell are you doing?" I ask.

"You've got to be really careful down here at the beach," he says. "Really, really careful."

Lenny lets a man with a heavy gray beard into the room. Lenny hands the man $200. The man hands Lenny an envelope. Then the man is gone. He has been in the apartment for only fifteen seconds. Neither he nor Lenny commented on the pistol.

Lenny opens the envelope and, standing over his glass-topped table, lets the pills drop on the surface. He gets forty pills for $200. He lines up all the "Lemmon" logos and peers under the table. "Goddammit," he says.

"The lines all go the same way?" I ask.

"Yeah. These are boots." Lenny picks up four of the pills and walks into the little bathroom. I can hear him run the water, hot water, because the pipes are squeaking and I can hear the hot-water heater turn on in the basement. "But they're not bad," he says. "Come in here."

Lenny holds the Quaaludes in one hand, the other testing the temperature of the heating water. "See," he says, laying three of the pills on the sink counter and holding out the remaining one to me. "It crumbles, just like a real one." Lenny pinches the corner of the big white pill, and the corner disintegrates into three or four small chunks and some powder. "A badly made boot is rock solid because it's full of impurities," Lenny explains. "This one's not real, but I can tell it's pretty close."

The water is hot enough now. Lenny takes a little from the tap and fills the bottom inch of a plastic drinking cup, the kind you get on airplanes. He dumps the crumbled pill and the three solid ones in the warm water. We watch them dissolve, turning the water a murky white. There are some lumps, but they get smaller as Lenny stirs the potion with his finger. Now there are no lumps. Lenny says, "Doesn't this look nice?" The doctors in Century City who took $400 a day to electro-convulse Lenny into being straight would be better able than I to say now nice it looks.

Daisy lies on the unmade bed and looks sad. She also looks well fed and brushed. Lenny loves his dog and his Panasonic.

Lenny goes to the refrigerator for a Diet Pepsi. Holding the plastic cup in one hand and a soda in the other, he says, "You've got to chase this stuff with something. You can mix it right in with orange juice, but I'm out of orange juice and Diet Pepsi is a great chaser. Not bad, anyway." He swallows the medicine first, making a face. A quick swallow of Diet Pepsi, a skip across the room, and Lenny is back in bed. Almost instantly, his hands have stopped shaking, a testament to the power of the drug in Lenny's mind.

In three minutes, he's not shaking at all. Lenny Brown is smiling and talking. He is finally bored by the television and asks me to turn it off. Lenny Brown feels great.

"I don't know where that guy gets his stuff," he says, "but it's great. He wants me to go in with him on the 'ludes, because I know some people. I could sell a few hundred back each month to the people in West Hollywood. It's tempting. It's sure tempting. Dealing. It can be a real trap. It's an easy way to make a lot of money. They're getting six bucks, six-fifty a pill now, for real ones. Ah," sighs Lenny, letting his head sink peacefully into a filthy pillow, "I guess it's just not worth it."

Of course, Lenny Brown would be dealing right now if he could get out of bed often enough. Soon he will be dealing, of that I am certain.

The water is still running in the bathroom. Lenny is in no condition to walk, so I go in and turn it off. The medicine chest is open. The top shelf is lined with jumbo—although empty—bottles of Quaaludes. I know they are Quaalude bottles because the label says in big red letters, "Methaqualone: 500—250 mg." If you could buy Quaaludes in the supermarket, this is what the jar would look like, if you were buying the Family Pak.

"Lenny," I ask, carrying one of the empty jars, "where the hell did you get this?" The jar clearly came directly from the pharmaceutical company. The company that made Quaaludes before Lemmon did—Rorer. The large quantity was not designed for individual consumption.

Lenny looks up at me. Moving his head is too big an effort, so he just slants his gaze toward the jar. Lenny smiles. "It's funny, isn't it?" he says. "That jar is why Lemmon took over from Rorer; making Quaaludes, I mean."

"I don't understand, Lenny."

"You don't?" Lenny sounds surprised. "It makes a lot of sense.

That bottle of five hundred you have there, well, that's how they come to the drugstores. I mean, you didn't think they came in little bottles of twenty-five, all ready to give to the people, did you?"

"I guess not."

"It's like anything else somebody sells," Lenny explains. "First you make the product, then you've gotta have distribution, right? Rorer would load up big trucks with bottles like that and send the trucks across the country, to everywhere, for delivery. Of course, they had other drugs in the trucks, too, but Quaaludes were what people were after."

"The trucks were hijacked?"

"That's right. What better way is there to get hold of a lot of 'ludes than hijacking a whole truck full of 'em? It got to the point where it wasn't worth it to Rorer to make 'em. They couldn't afford the insurance, man. Just too expensive."

Lenny's eyelids droop, his breathing becomes heavier. There is still a trace of a smile lingering on his face. It is a satisfied smile that means he has just explained something important to me. Now Lenny's eyes are tiny slits, but that is not because he has fallen asleep. It is because Lenny is very, very high. He looks peaceful, almost beatific.

"That's pretty interesting," Lenny says after a while. His words have become slurred.

"You mean about the trucks, Lenny?" I ask, because when Lenny is high his train of thought is often hard to follow. I need to make sure.

"Yeah," he says. "And the insurance. You wanna know why Rorer was able to give up the manufacture of Quaaludes without worrying about losing too much money?"

"Tell me," I say.

"Did you bring me the Diet Pepsi in the little bottles?" Lenny asks. I pick up the bottle that's resting perhaps eight inches from his right hand and hand it to him.

"Oh, yeah," he says, "we were talking about Rorer, right?"

"That's right."

"Well, first of all, they made a ton of money selling out to Lemmon. But that's not why they didn't care. You want to know why they didn't care?"

"Why, Lenny?"

"Because," says Lenny Brown, conspiratorially, "because Rorer makes something else, too. Something that coins money for them. Something that no one ever steals, because everyone has it in the first place. You know what it is?"

"No."

"Rorer's got the franchise," says Lenny, "on Valium. Just what do you figure that's worth?"

Something catches my eye, and I look over on the floor, to my left. A huge roach is crawling into an old, crumb-filled bag of Doritos. Somewhere else in the apartment the roach has picked up a small dust ball and hooked it through his antenna like a little hat.

"It's got to be worth a lot of money, Lenny."

Lenny chuckles. "You bet. A lot."

The telephone rings. It rings five times before Lenny appears to notice it, six when I ask him if he wants me to pick it up.

"Yeah," says Lenny. "That would be great."

I lift the receiver, say hello, and hear a click. Someone has hung up. I tell Lenny.

"You know," he says, "I should really get one of those answering machines. That way I could tell who was calling and if I wanted to pick up."

"That's a waste of money," I say. Lenny just smiles. I can tell him the truth when he's had a few 'ludes. I can say anything, because he's not really there.

"You see Linda anymore?" he asks out of nowhere. "If you do, please tell her I said hello. Is she still dancing a lot? Still with that doctor guy?"

"Yes," I say. "She's doing just fine. She's worried about you, though. She asks about you all the time."

"Next time you see her, be sure to say hello," he repeats. Lenny Brown is talking about his ex-wife, whose abrupt departure recently meant about as much to him as cutting off my head would mean to me, and still he talks about her as if she were a distant relative. *These days.* "Tell her I'm really glad she's doing OK. Tell her I'm doing great, too. I'm going to get back into real-estate syndication pretty soon. The market's lousy right now, but I'll be back in it when the market picks up. It's those damn interest rates."

"It's not the damn interest rates," I say. The methaquaalone coursing through Lenny's blood does not permit him to hear the disappointment in my voice. He just smiles at me. Lenny is way off in the ozone somewhere, where none of it has happened, where life is still *as it was*, where he still has all the ambition, all the drive, the money, the wife, the edge. When he's had the Quaaludes, the Vitamin-Q, the gorilla biscuits, the disco wafers, the Sopors, he's where the dream of *what was* and *what could be*, if there were a miracle, are both the same.

Lenny's face, *these days:* it is rapt. It is still a handsome face, with a straight nose and a high forehead and a cleft chin. He also has a cut on his cheek, where he fell down when he was trying to go to the deli to get a sandwich a few nights ago. Lenny's cuts take a long time to heal *these days*. Lenny gazes off toward the blank, cold Panasonic, but his brown eyes do not see a thing. He's taken four Quaaludes and is in the part of that high where he sees absolutely nothing. It is as if he decided simply to *give away* an hour of his life. There is no point in talking to him for at least another half hour.

"Lenny," I say out loud to myself, "I'm going for a walk." I am not sure if I am just going out. I might go home.

If Lenny wakes up and I'm not there, he will assume I said good-bye.

I walk south along the now deserted boardwalk. To my right, about fifty feet out on the beach, an old man in a camouflage suit combs the sand with a metal detector. To my left is a condominium building rising above a liquor store. If I remember correctly, Lenny was once "putting together" a deal to build condominiums at Venice Beach. It was absolutely guaranteed, beyond the shadow of a doubt, to make Lenny Brown a millionaire. It never happened. Not even close. I wonder if any of Lenny's deals did fall into place. Maybe in Reseda or West Covina there is a shopping center with a "7-11," a real-estate office, a gift shop, and a Thai restaurant which is a monument to Lenny as he once was.

I walk back to Lenny's, alone with my thoughts and a stiff evening breeze off the ocean. The breeze blows bad thoughts away.

A single bare yellow light bulb lights up Lenny's "kitchenette." It's a closet, really, with just a two-burner stove and a sink and a half-sized refrigerator stuck in it. Lenny is up now, in the kitchen, whistling the final number from *Evita*. He is still pretty stoned, so he cannot whistle very well.

"Hey," says Lenny cheerfully. "Have a seat. I'm making coffee here. Great coffee." I sit down at the small white wooden table, scarred with cigarettes and circled with the sticky bottoms of Diet Pepsis. Lenny sets a cup and saucer in front of me. "Oh," he says, "you're going to need a spoon." Lenny hands me a spoon. I look at the face of the spoon and decide that I will take my coffee black.

"Goddammit it!" Lenny screams. He has bashed his knee against the top edge of the mini-refrigerator. It is not the first time. "This place is just too goddam small," Lenny says, "even for one person."

The rest of the Quaaludes are still on the glass-topped table. Lenny sees me looking at them, so he looks, too. "If you take those all the time," Lenny says, "you can really get in trouble. So," he continues, "Linda's really worried about me? There's no reason to. What does she say?"

After taking four 'ludes, Lenny often returns to a seminormal manner. He asks a lot of questions and does not care about the answers. The pills have distracted him, confused him with their power.

"Linda wonders if you're all right, Lenny," I said.

"You know what Linda's always wanted?" Lenny dumps a spoonful of coffee crystals into my grimy cup. "Linda's always wanted one of those new Rolex watches. You know, the First Lady model, for women. It's really a beautiful watch. There's one that mixes silver and gold on the face, but I think what she really wants is the all-gold one, eighteen-karat. There's a place down here that's got the dealership. I've done some favors for the owner. I can get one at a pretty good price."

Lenny takes my cup from the table to the sink and fills it from the tap. The water is not quite hot enough to dissolve the coffee. Lenny stirs it with his other spoon to get rid of the lumps. He hands the cup back to me. I take a couple of careful sips. I will have to tell Tony, the captain at La Scala, how Lenny takes his coffee *these days*.

Lenny watches me as I drink. "Pretty good," he says. "And there's no caffeine in this stuff, either. Caffeine," Lenny says, "can really fuck you up."

"Tastes fine to me, Lenny," I say. "Aren't you having any?"

"No," says Lenny, pressing his hands to his temples. "I'm getting a little bit of a headache. It's the smog. I'm sure of it. They tell you it's not so bad down here at the beach, but that's a joke. The smog is just as bad, it only smells better. I've got to lie down for a minute.

I follow Lenny into the bedroom proper. We assume our original positions. Lenny clicks on the Panasonic with his remote control. It's a new show, one I've never seen. It has girls in boarding-school uniforms. "Facts of Life," another money machine for Norman Lear.

"It's a very clever show," Lenny says. "What do you think about the watch?"

"I've seen the ads in the *New Yorker*," I say. "It's a very beautiful watch, Lenny."

"It costs three grand," Lenny says, "but it's worth it. I can just see her face when she opens that box. Wow. Can you see her face?"

"Lenny," I say, "it's a wonderful gift."

"You bet," he says happily. "You bet. An extremely wonderful gift."

We watch a little more of the show. From where I am sitting I can see the physical and emotional cycles in Lenny. They are starting all over again. His face falls like a time-lapse photograph of wilting flowers. His breathing becomes regular, rhythmic. His eyes look at the television, yet they lack any focus.

"I'll tell her you're going to get her one," I say. "I'll tell Linda."

"Get her one of what?" Lenny asks, getting up for just one more Quaalude that he'll take straight, without dissolving it in warm water.

There is no point in talking to Lenny now. I sit in a dusty arm-chair, and I think about life for Lenny and Linda *as it was.* A few minutes pass and I say good-bye.

"Thanks for visiting me," Lenny says, back in bed now. "I hope you'll excuse me if I don't get up. I've really got a terrific headache."

"That's OK, Lenny," I say. "No problem. Take care of yourself."

Lenny raises his hand to stop my departure. "Listen," he says, "if you see Linda, tell her that I've joined this group down here that's taking care of lost dogs and rabbits. For some reason, there are a lot of rabbits that get lost down here. Anyway, I'm working with them. I work at the shelter, cleaning up and feeding the dogs once a week. That's really important to me, to get out to do that. I hope you'll tell that to Linda, let her know I'm keeping up my end for the dogs."

"I'll tell her," I say. Lenny is not lying. He loves lost dogs. He will even forgo 'ludes for the few hours while he works with abandoned, terrified dogs. Lenny is like a pelican. He would actually tap open his chest, or open his veins and give his heart's blood, to keep poor lost dogs from feeling overwhelmed and hysterical with fear. "I'll tell her," I say again, and then I leave.

On the ride back to Hollywood I listen to the radio. I try every station. Nothing sounds good. *These days.*

Lenny Brown. Driving home, I thought a lot about Lenny Brown. He has come a long way since that day when he walked into my office at the *Wall Street Journal* to ask me if I wanted to invest $500,000 in a real-estate syndication. He was wrong then and he's wrong now, but there is a lot of pain between those two mistakes.

Because I love Lenny, because I see him as a dear, lost soul, just like the lost dogs he has befriended in recent years, saw him like that years before, it hurts like the cut of a knife to see the way Lenny lives *these days.* But as I look back on it now, perhaps it was always inevitable from the very beginning.

THE DREAM BEGINS

In the spring of 1976 I was the only member of the *Wall Street Journal*'s editorial-page staff who had had any graduate training in economics. I suppose that was why I was rigorously discouraged from writing anything about economics. While the other editorial writers sat at their gray metal desks chortling about the possibility of New York City going bankrupt—something they were all rooting for—I sat at my gray metal desk making appointments to interview Ringo Starr. The *Wall Street Journal*'s editorial page at that time was to supply-side economics what New Orleans was to jazz. From those metal cubicles came the philosophy that would rock the world and help to make an actor President. But I was not part of the supply-side club. So I watched Arthur Laffer coming and going, but paid no mind.

In lieu of writing about the subject I knew best, I wrote about the subject I liked best: popular culture. Off I would go to concerts by Big Al Greene, disco parties for the BeeGees, smoky dinners with The Manhattan Transfer, afternoons watching soap operas on videotape monitors at ABC. Out would come columns explaining where America was going by reference to the signposts of rock lyrics, plots of "Mary Tyler Moore," heroes and villains of movies.

I was also assigned to distribute book reviews to the hordes of desperate writers who wanted to see their names in print. One day, while I looked at a particularly promising letter of inquiry from the typical *Wall Street Journal* reader, a retired investment banker in Pelham Bay, I was interrupted by a loud guffaw from the man who sat at the next desk.

"And can you believe it?" this man shouted into his telephone, "Ford says we should cut the depreciation allowance by two point seven percent, when even Bill Simon says it should be cut by at the most two point five percent!" Then he fell into gales of laughter.

That was a standard conversation—or half of a conversation—at the *Wall Street Journal*'s editorial page. They were a smart bunch, but I never could understand why they were so interested in taxes.

I went back to my stack of books, hoping against hope to find one with dirty pictures. The telephone at my desk rang. It was Johnny, the elderly Irishman who guarded the fifth-floor reception room against the assaults of any Keynesians who might have wandered in off Cortlandt Street. "Ben," he said in his raspy voice, "there's a gentleman here to see you."

Frankly, I lived in dread of such a call. My columns were always infuriating people. I could easily see a fan of "Ryan's Hope" coming to kill me because I had not raved about it. In addition, there were simply too many crazy people in this world. "I'm not expecting anyone," I said.

There was a pause while I could hear Johnny interrogating my visitor. That was the first time I had ever heard Lenny Brown's voice. It was a deep, confident voice, laced with tolerant amusement of Johnny's questions. It might have been a local TV commentator's voice. I could not hear what the voice said. In fact, I could hardly hear what anyone else said. My neighbor was now laughing hysterically about a proposal for taxation of foreign dividends, blocking out every other sound.

I could barely hear Johnny say, "The gentleman says he's from your bank."

Perfect. I did not ever balance my checkbook. Perhaps I was so overdrawn that the bank had sent a human representative to arrest me. It was possible. Manufacturers Hanover was right across the street. They might do anything.

I went out the long corridor to the elevators. There was Johnny, small and neat in his gray elevator starter's uniform, his cigar in his teeth. Next to him was a smiling, tall man wearing a well-cut suit—Paul Stuart, I guessed—of brown wool, elegant loafers, a respectable rep tie, and an obvious Brooks Brothers pink shirt. He had a handsome face with good, strong features; a healthy tan; intelligent brown eyes; and a sharp, inquisitive-looking nose. He stuck out his hand to me as if he had known me for years and Johnny was a fool to have been so protective.

A smarter person would have spotted the con a mile away, but if I were that smart, I would not have been at the *Wall Street Journal* at a gray metal desk.

"Hi," he said, "how've you been keeping yourself?"

"I'm sorry," I said. "I don't remember where we met."

"We can talk about all of it. May I come to your office?" he asked, starting down the hall. Once we had turned the corner, he stuck out his hand again and said, "How the hell are you? I'm Lenny Brown."

"Are you from Manufacturers Hanover Trust?" I asked. I steered him toward a conference room. No sense humiliating myself in front of the other staffers.

"Oh, hell, no," he said. "Where'd you get that idea?"

"I thought you told that to Johnny," I said.

"I don't know where he got that idea," he answered. "I told him I'm from Equity Appreciation Associates, and maybe he got the idea that it was a bank."

In the conference room, I studied him more carefully. He sat on one of the uncomfortable swivel chairs where the week's editorials were parceled out on Monday mornings, just under a framed *Wall Street Journal* from December 8, 1941. ("U.S. Well Stocked With Far Eastern Commodities," said a subhead.) He still looked handsome. But on closer examination under the pitiless fluorescent lights, he looked worried. He was far too eager-looking to have come from any bank, far too tight around the mouth. His knuckles were too white.

"You know," I said, "I think you probably want someone from the news side. I mainly write columns about television. I think you want someone from the business side. Maybe on the sixth floor. Are you looking for a story?"

"No way," he said, smiling broadly. "You're the one I want to talk to. I have a big favor for you."

That was when even I started to get worried.

"If you will listen to me for a few minutes, I think we can save you at least two hundred fifty thousand dollars on your this year's income tax. That's a nice piece of change," he said cheerfully.

"I think you must be making a joke," I said. "Did Larry send you?"

"No way," he said again. "I'm serious. I'm talking about a highly leveraged investment in cattle-feeding programs. The write-off is four to one in the first year alone. That means you put up one hundred twenty-five thousand, then throw it against unearned income; you can get a write-off of half a million against seventy percent, which would give you a tax savings of more than a quarter million. More like three hundred fifty thousand." He winked at me. "All perfectly legal. All approved by the IRS. Perfectly kosher."

I started to laugh. "Look," I said, "you must be kidding me. I earned twenty-three thousand two hundred dollars last year. This is a newspaper. I'm a lowly guy here."

"Ben," he said, "I know all about that. I happen to be talking about the interest income from the money your father gave you."

"My father is a professor," I said. "You're talking way out of our league."

"Your father isn't Howard Stein, from the Dreyfus Fund?" he asked.

"Oh, God," I said. "You're so wrong. Where the hell did you get that idea?" I was starting to laugh a lot now.

"A girl you went out with is a friend of my wife's," he said. "She told me about you. She said your father was real famous and had something to do with money. I put two and two together." He shook his head and laughed. "I knew I should have spent more time on arithmetic. I'm going to have to go back to third grade now and really give my teacher hell."

But for some reason, this mistake, this failure, did not seem to make Lenny sad. Far from it. Instead, he looked relieved, as if he no longer had to make a sale he probably was not going to make, anyway. His face softened and became positively boyish.

"You saved me a lot of trouble by not jerking me along," he said after he laughed. "I'll buy you lunch. Maybe you know someone who can use a three-hundred-fifty-thousand-dollar tax shelter."

We ate at Harry's American Bar, right in the old American Stock Exchange Building. The only good thing on the menu was liver. The salt sticks were also good, but they were not on the menu.

"I'll tell you, man," he said, "I'm batting a thousand on these tax shelters, so far. O for five. Maybe that's batting zero." I should have known by then that Lenny had trouble adding things up. "I think I'm going to have to find a new scam. The thing is, though, if I can just sell one of these damned things, I get five percent right off the top. That means if you had bought in, I would have gotten six thousand, maybe a little more. Just for one afternoon's work, or one morning's work."

"But you haven't sold any yet," I said. "That's the problem."

"I'm talking about how it's going to be," Lenny said. "I'm not talking about the way it is now. It's always rough at first. Especially because my bosses don't really send me out to the best gigs. They send me out to drum up business any way I can. That's why I make these dumb fucking mistakes."

"Maybe the whole line of work isn't right for you. Maybe you shouldn't be a salesman," I said as I ate my fourth salt stick.

Lenny shook his head emphatically. His face started to color. "Let me tell you something, man," he said. "The fastest way to make really major dollars in this world is to sell things. The guys you see who're twenty-five years old and driving around in Excaliburs are the guys who sell things. I know guys who aren't even twenty-five who sell things like fucking time shares in condominiums, and those guys are making a fortune, man. A real fortune." He stuffed a shaved carrot into his mouth and looked around the room, as if an unknown enemy lurked there who might be trying to keep him from being a successful salesman.

"I just think it's hard to go around peddling things to people," I said. "That's all. It really hurts your feelings when you get turned down."

"I'm hip," Lenny said. "But that's the price you pay. Sometimes you get your feelings hurt. That doesn't matter. What matters is how much money you bring home. That's all anyone gives a goddam about in this world, and you know it."

"I'm sorry," I said. "I don't know it and I don't believe it." Lenny did not contradict me. He obviously thought I was making a joke.

His point was so obviously true, at least to him, that it did not really brook any questioning. What a world to live in, I thought. A world in which no one cares about anything but how much money you bring home. It's almost like being in a prison camp. Worse, maybe. Some people eventually get out of prison camps.

I thought that Lenny Brown had better learn some new rules or maybe some new games, or else he was going to be in a lot of trouble. The world rarely affords much comfort to people who think that all that matters is how much money you bring home.

On the other hand, I could see exactly Lenny's point. I had just come to the *Wall Street Journal* from a political job which had once seemed secure and prestigious, but which overnight had become nonexistent and shameful. I had no money. If I had had money at the time I lost my political job, I might well have spent fewer sleepless nights in a rented house in Georgetown.

More important, even before the debacle at the Nixon White House, I had often felt that no one in the world valued anything except money. I had seen incredibly brilliant professors and scholars humiliated by manufacturers of paper cups who could not form sentences. I had seen wives of Cabinet officials toadying to millionaires in the folding-box business. I could definitely see Lenny's point. But I liked to think that there was a point beyond that point, which was that even if you did have money, there would always be people with more, and then they would humiliate you and make you crazy. I also considered myself an artist of sorts, and so, for reasons of basic self-worth, I had to at least pretend to myself that money was not the value in life that was universally accepted. (I'm not certain I believe that any longer, but the conversation with Lenny took place before I lived in Los Angeles.)

Enough of me was speaking through Lenny, though, so that I felt a certain empathy. Lenny was saying what I thought but could not bring myself to admit so openly. That crucial basis for friendship was laid down immediately. As Lenny and I traveled farther in life, the pattern recurred endlessly. Lenny would live out and say what I only thought or feared. Lenny was like a feral Ben Stein, without the repression or the care to stay above water. Put more precisely, Lenny was the most basic me, and so I had to like him at first and then love him.

Lenny and I chewed our liver, watched the brokers file in and out, talking about tennis and private schools. Lenny told me that he came from a bad neighborhood in Brooklyn called Red Hook, which was mostly Italian, but a few Jews lived there, too. I didn't learn until much later whether Lenny was Jewish or Italian himself, or some other "race" altogether. Sometimes he would tell people he was Jewish, and other times he would tell people he was a *paisano*. Lenny had been a good student at his high school. He also got into a lot of fights. "I was never afraid to fight, man," he said. "Even with the spades. They're tough, but if you smash one in the face, he's going to hurt just like everyone else. If you kick him in the guts, he's going down just like everybody else."

Lenny told me that he had gotten a scholarship to N.Y.U. so that he could get the hell out of Red Hook. "All the kids I went to high school with wound up in jail or getting killed in Vietnam," he said. "That ain't for me. No way."

"I'm hip," I said. He was already starting to influence me.

He had studied business at N.Y.U., but with a minor in English. "I love to read, man," he said. "There's a lot of people who say it's a waste of time, but I love to read."

Lenny read every one of the top five books on the fiction list of best sellers in the *New York Times*. He did that on a continuing basis, he told me, because he might discover a story idea, which he could sell to a network for a TV movie. "Mucho buckos," he said.

Plus, Lenny just plain liked words. He was fascinated with corporate names. "Look at Consolidated Rock Products Industries," he said. "It sounds solid. It should be selling for a lot. It never moves. Then look at Litton. It sounds as if it could be blown away by a breeze, but its stock is selling for twenty times earnings."

I thought that Lenny was a pleasant—although driven—breath of poetry blowing into Harry's American Bar. Naturally, no one paid any attention to him except me, and I am a notorious waster of time.

During college, Lenny had worked part-time selling shirts at Bloomingdale's main store on Lexington Avenue. "That was really an education," he said. "These guys would come in and buy ten shirts at a time at thirty bucks a pop. They didn't even think twice about it. A lot of them were fags. They just plopped down their credit cards and had the shirts delivered. Three hundred bucks for shirts at one pop. And that's not counting the tax, which is another twenty-five or thirty bucks." At the time, Lenny was getting paid four dollars per hour, or enough to buy one shirt per day.

"I copped a lot of shirts, though," Lenny said. "I guarantee you that I was never short of shirts. Never. The store just assumed they were stolen, so what the hell. It isn't like Bloomingdale's can't afford it."

Lenny did not see why he should not be able to have as many shirts as all those rich assholes who came into the store with their fag boyfriends. In this world, you take what you want. "There was this great movie," he said. *"Murder Incorporated*. It was about Louis Lepke Buchalter. In this one scene he's telling someone to move in on someone else's territory. The guy he's talking to has all these excuses. So Louis Lepke just grabs the guy by the shoulders and he says, 'You have arms? You take.' And that's what it's all about."

When Lenny told me these stories, these fables with their maxims for his life, he pronounced them with a certain wild bravado. He was a child telling of the exploits of the Lone Ranger or the Cisco Kid. There was something touching about the seriousness with which he told the stories of his toughness and his role models of ruthless piracy. I have found it to be an inflexible rule that those who talk most about being tough are the softest, the most vulnerable, and those who talk most about being reasonable and getting hurt are the toughest. I do not remember Lyndon Johnson ever talking publicly about what a tough sonofabitch he was, or Leonid Brezhnev, either. But Lenny did, even though he had those soft, frightened brown eyes. Lenny, even then, was a timid child raising his courage by telling himself tales about bravery, a giver trying to steel himself with stories about taking.

From that early meeting with Lenny, whose life was to move so far away from Harry's American Bar, I could see something fundamentally askew about Lenny, and that also made me like him. Like me, he literally did not fit in with himself. Not only was Lenny in an entire world in which he was uncomfortable—the world of making money—he was also a lost soul drifting alone within his own personality. He was constantly having to tell himself to be tough, to go fight, to make money, to take, when what he really liked was to have a friend to talk to, to think about how words sound, to look at life and see what made it work. Instead, he was out on the street hustling, selling tax shelters. He was not only the square peg in the round hole, but also a peg which did not know how it should be shaped. And again, there was enough similarity between Lenny and me to make me feel something for him. After all, I was on a crowded, dusty street in lower Manhattan when I wanted to be in a field in Colorado, or somewhere where people talked about flowers instead of about taxes. More importantly, I was there voluntarily, knowing it was not what I wanted, a sure sign of confusion about self.

From the work at Bloomingdale's, Lenny learned that he wanted to be able to walk in off Fifty-ninth Street, plunk down a credit card, and have ten shirts delivered, without having even to think about how much they cost. "If you have to worry about how much every little thing costs, you might as well forget it and just stay home and eat TV dinners." Still, when the check came, he held it for a minute and asked if I had an expense account at the *Wall Street Journal* that would take care ot it. "I'm just curious," he said.

"I'm afraid not," I said. "We split it."

"No way," he said. "I'll take care of it. Let Equity Appreciation Associates pick it up."

As we walked up Cortlandt Street back to my office, Lenny asked me if I were married. I told him I was not. "I am," he said. "I'm married to someone wonderful. That's the only thing in my life that's perfect right now. My wife. I was really, really lucky to get her. We'll have you over for dinner and then you can see. A lot of people say she looks like Anouk Aimée. I think she does, too. I don't know how I ever got her."

Lenny said he was going to catch a cab, but he walked off in the direction of the subway.

About a week later, Pat, one of the two stalwart secretaries at the *Wall Street Journal* editorial page, interrupted my article on "Laverne and Shirley" to tell me that Lenny Brown was calling. He got on the phone and invited me to dinner with him and his wife Linda. "I want you to see this very special little Italian place on the East Side. Not many people know about it. The owner doesn't even have a sign out in front. He has to know you personally to let you in. He doesn't even like for me to bring anybody besides Linda. That's the kind of place it is. But I swear to you, it has the best saltimbocca in New York, and it's really cheap. If you were Jackie Onassis, you wouldn't get in there if the owner didn't like you. But I did him a couple of favors with people in the trucking business, so we're buddies. How about Tuesday night?"

I have often wondered why many people feel it necessary to talk about their friends in the trucking business or the linen-supply business or the magazine-delivery business. In those days, Lenny was the first. But as I have moved around in life, gone from the library into the casino, I have met more and more people who have done favors for Meyer Lansky's lawyer or know Frank Sinatra's accountant or are owed a few by someone very high up at Caesar's. Once again, I have the feeling that the real *mafiosi* boast about knowing professors of Renaissance Literature at Princeton.

I Stigmati was not worth knowing about. It was simply another two-bit neighborhood restaurant in Yorkville. The tablecloths were dirty. There was no sign of any boss who knew Lenny. The waiter was a surly Puerto Rican. The saltimbocca was one desiccated bone with a little tasteless sauce thrown over it.

But Linda was really a prize. She was an Italianate-looking woman with jet-black hair, a wonderful figure, and dark blue eyes. She had a mischievous look about her eyes. Her nose was thin, long, and upturned. Her lips always pouted, except when she laughed.

Her skin was absolutely smooth, like the marble of a statue. I thought Lenny was pretty lucky to have her.

She told me about her life. She had been born to a Czech father and an Italian mother in Marlboro, Massachusetts. Amazingly enough in this day and age, she grew up on a dairy farm. She hated the Berkshires, though, with their interminable cloudiness and cold. "Plus," she said, "there was no cable TV, no decent restaurants, no friends." All there was for Linda was the ballet at Tanglewood for her to drive to during the summer, and the little ballet studio above the pizza place in Marlboro where she had her lesson every day after school.

"You can imagine what it was like to love ballet and live in western Massachusetts. It would have been a lot better if I had liked painting landscapes."

So off she went to New York University, where this really funny guy sat behind her in Freshman English. "And you know," she said, "he always had the right answers for everything. The teacher would give him a poem to interpret, something really hard by Emily Dickinson, and he would know what the poem was about even better than the teacher did. I always thought Lenny should have become an English teacher."

Linda Brown looked at Lenny as if he were a god and she were a temple virgin. Not too many men get wives who look at them that way.

Lenny laughed. He held his wineglass in his right hand. He held that glass with a particular gentleness, like a ballet dancer holding the prima ballerina or a hound dog holding an egg. A dog will never crush an egg in its mouth. It will hold that egg firmly, but without ever breaking it, until you tell the dog to give you back the egg. Even the most untrained dog knows to do that instinctively. That was how Lenny held his wineglass. As if it might break if he did not take care of it. But while he held the glass gently, he laughed harshly. "An English teacher! No way. Those guys are lucky if they can afford Pintos. I want a Mercedes," he said. "I could never live on that kind of money. If it did pay better, though," he said, "I could do a helluva good job at it. I'd like it, too." That was the only time I ever heard Lenny express genuine enthusiasm for work, entirely apart from money.

Lenny listened to every word Linda said. Linda listened to every word Lenny said. I thought that Lenny might have terrible taste in restaurants, but he had found a wonderful wife.

We walked back to Lenny and Linda's apartment. It was in a tall white-brick building on the corner of Eighty-seventh and York. The apartment building had a Waldbaum's on the ground floor. "I started out slicing lox at Waldbaum's after school when I was fourteen years old," Lenny said. "That was my first job. It took me about a month to get the smell out of my hands after I quit."

Lenny and Linda had a one-bedroom apartment on the fifth floor of the building. If you craned your neck, you could see out to the East River. The apartment had some nice features. It had modular furniture, which meant that the sofa and the chair looked as if each had been sliced from the same long roll of foam rubber. It also had a VCR stashed right under a twenty-one-inch Sony, which I thought was pretty fancy. Lenny had a Sansui amplifier and Bose speakers hooked up to a Sony turntable. It was so powerful that the floor shook when he turned it up. The lights dimmed when it hit a bass note. There was a series of Lichtenstein prints on the walls. The subject was a fighter plane shooting down another fighter plane. The triptych was filled with explosions and fireballs. It was entitled "As I Opened Fire."

Linda told Lenny and me to just sit down and relax, and she would make us some espresso. They also had an espresso machine. "Lenny gets me everything I want," Linda said. I thought she was a happy woman. It is rare for a woman who is so good-looking to be so devoted to a man.

"See," Lenny said, "this is a pretty nice place. When people from Red Hook come to see me, they can't believe I have a place like this. I mean they can't fucking believe it. But this is just the beginning. Someday this place is going to be the place where our maid lives."

"Oh, Lenny," Linda said from the kitchen. "I like this place. It's really a lot nicer than I ever thought I'd live in. It really is."

Plus, the apartment was really convenient to Linda's job. She worked as a typist at a law firm in Rockefeller Center. She just had to take a crosstown bus and then one subway, and she was there. It was even more convenient to the dance studio, which was right there on Eighty-sixth street and Third Avenue. She went there five times a week. Lenny looked proud when she talked about her dancing. He looked embarrassed when she talked about working as a typist.

"You won't be doing that much longer," he said. "It's just temporary, until things get better at Equity Appreciation Associates."

Lenny had worked for a lot of people since he had gotten out of school nine years ago. He had been a customers' man at Bache, but that fell through because who was buying stock in 1974? Then he had been a real-estate salesman for Douglas, Elliman, but the co-op market was strictly from hunger in those days. Then he had worked as a fund raiser for some mail-order company whose name he could not even remember. That was how much he hated it. And there were a few others, too. In the meantime, Linda worked as a typist. She was far too tall to dance professionally. "My boobs are too big, too," she said, blushing as she said it. So she worked at a few different typing jobs and danced in the evenings until Lenny got moving. This time, he was sure, he had finally found the people who thought big enough. "The guys who own the company are taking a couple of million a year out of it every year," he said.

"I understand," I said. On one wall of Lenny and Linda's living room there was a bookshelf. Most of the books were about astrology. But there were also several books about making money by buying apartment buildings with no money down. I did not see any books about taxes.

"See," he said, "that kind of thing doesn't mean anything to you. It doesn't, does it?" He looked at me almost belligerently.

"What kind of thing are you talking about?" I asked.

"Going out and hustling and making some money," he said. "You couldn't care less about that. It's like something you never have to worry about."

I wondered if Lenny had drunk too many martinis.

"I'm sure I worry about money just as much as you do," I said. "Probably more."

"Oh, you may worry about it," he said. "But you know that there are a lot of backstops. Like you know that if you start to fall down into the well, there are a lot of slats across the well that'll keep you from falling too far."

"I don't know what you mean," I said. "I'm sure I make less money than you do. Probably a lot less."

Lenny and I had this kind of conversation frequently. It was his oblique, almost Japanese, way of insuring that we were still on the same wavelength.

"I saw a really funny thing on the bus today," Linda said. "A man was trying to get a French horn onto the bus."

Lenny ignored her. "See, you've got that professor father, and he probably knows lots of important people. And then you've got the crew at the *Wall Street Journal*. Once you've worked there, there's practically nothing you can't do. So you've got this like net under you, just to protect you. So you shouldn't fall too far."

I shook my head. "I don't know, Lenny," I said. "I think it's up to us all alone, really." By now, this was all rote for me and him.

"And the bus driver wanted him to pay another fifty cents for the French horn," Linda said.

"No, but I couldn't get shit from my parents," Lenny said. "First of all, my father doesn't work at all anymore. He was a printer, but he hurt his back and now he's on disability. And my mother's a secretary at the headquarters of the ILGWU. So how're they going to help me if I'm in trouble?"

"There's all kinds of help," I said.

"I mean with money, man. Who's going to help me with money?"

Linda looked so sad that I thought her whole body might dissolve into one large sob. Lenny caught that look and got up. He put his arm around her shoulders. She knew it was all a routine, too, and still it saddened her profoundly.

"I don't care," he said. "Fuck 'em all. As long as I have Linda, I don't really need anyone else." He had delivered the entire dialogue in a tone which was not hostile to me at all but expressed resigned and not yet complete disappointment in the world at large.

Linda then delivered the final line of the formulistic drama.

She pulled her face together and smiled. "So the man with the French horn said he would play a concert for everyone, instead. And he did. All the way across Eighty-sixth Street."

I saw Lenny and Linda every two weeks or so during that time right after I met them. Lenny always had a new secret restaurant that no one else knew about. We would get into subways and taxicabs and travel all around New York, sometimes even into Brooklyn, to find restaurants that were never worth the trip. Kampuchean food, Chilean food, Turkish food. Always, the host would never let us in except that Lenny had done a very special favor for him when some tough guys were threatening his restaurant. Never a sign of the host. Often, there was no else in the restaurant. Lenny would talk the entire evening about how he had put it to some rude prospect; about how he had really shown someone on the street who bumped into him; about how he had told off a sarcastic waiter at Mercurio's; about how his bosses still were not thinking big enough, particularly about him, were still giving him little piss-ant assignments, making him drum up his own customers, when all the time they had these lists of multimillionaires they were just using for themselves.

Lenny spoke of a world which unrelentingly pressed down upon him its threats, its dangers, its belittlement, its insults, its mockery. He spoke of a man-child who struggled constantly to keep from being buried under the weight of cruelty that rained upon him every day. It did not take me long to realize that Lenny made up most of his stories about threatening people with broken beer bottles and drawing a Walther PPK on a black man in an alley. But made up or not, the stories were the epic of Lenny's labors, day by day. And, again, on a certain level, I saw my own face in Lenny's mirror.

At a certain time in May, it became clear to me that Lenny either had been fired or was about to be fired. His conversations with me became far more frequent. He talked of feeling that he was at a dead end, that he was much bigger than his job, that he would never get anywhere until he had "room to maneuver," as one of his favorite phrases went. He stopped telling me incidents of work and instead told me about how he had perceived certain social facts in television game shows. Perhaps I could get him a few columns at the *Journal*. Or maybe I could get him at least a mention in one of my columns. That would help him a lot in unspecified ways.

One day he asked me to meet him at a restaurant near Times Square. By a mercy of life, I have forgotten which one. He told me that I could do him a great favor. "Do you think you could write something for your column about a massage parlor? Maybe mention one by name and say how good you thought it was?"

"I would have to think real hard about what kind of an angle that would be, Lenny," I said. "It's not the usual kind of thing for the *Journal*."

After lunch, he took me to the massage parlor. It was a converted town house with red flocked wallpaper, heavy metal doors, and thin men with thin leather jackets running the front desk. Lenny and the men knew each other. But it was hardly a relationship of equals. Lenny was obviously trying to curry favor with the owners by bringing me around. He arranged for me to talk to two of the masseuses. They were glazed-eyed overweight blond girls who told me it was their job to give men "sexual relief."

Outside, on Forty-eighth Street, I told Lenny that it would be impossible to write anything about the massage parlor.

"It would mean a lot to me, pal," he said. "A real lot."

"I'm sorry," I said.

"They were going to give me twenty-five hundred to get an article in. I'd be glad to give you half," he said.

"I'm sorry," I said.

A few days after that, Lenny got the break that would alter his life. Apparently he was meeting a group of real-estate investors to pitch himself to them as a salesman for a shopping center in northwestern Connecticut. He went in looking supertweedy, in a new suit from Chipp. He gave them his all-out best pitch about how qualified he was, how he could sell snowshoes to penguins, and they turned him down flat.

But one of the men came over to talk to Lenny when the meeting was over. His name was Max Sherman. He was a heavyset guy with a turquoise and silver buckle on his cowboy belt. He was very heavy into shopping centers in Los Angeles and north San Diego and Orange counties in southern California. He told Lenny that the problem with people in southern California was that they got a few million dollars and then they got soft. He needed a man who was hungry down to his socks, a man who wouldn't quit after he made a couple of million dollars.

He and Lenny went for a drink at a bar on Fifty-seventh Street. Max Sherman told Lenny that his accountants, who were also the accountants to some of the biggest names in Hollywood, had assured him that he could work out an investor-participation scheme with a difference. The difference was that the investors could see current income which would not be taxable, plus they would get a share of an investment tax credit. I did not understand how it worked, and I suspect Lenny did not, either. But he acted as if that kind of arrangement were second nature to him.

Max told Lenny that a man who knew taxes the way he did and knew how to sell the way he did would make two million dollars pretty damn quick. "But the thing I want to be pretty sure of, boychik," he said, "is that if I bring you out there and get you started, that once you've made your first million in cash that you don't just lie by your pool all day and forget about your pal Max who first discovered you."

Lenny assured Max that even if he made fifty million dollars in syndications, he would still be a salesman first, last, and always.

"It's in my blood, man," he said. "I'm not the kind of guy who likes to just sit around. I like the selling more than the money."

Max said he would call Lenny as soon as he got back to Los Angeles. Now, Lenny didn't just fall off the truck. He knew the score. When Max said he'd call, Lenny figured it was all a jerk-off. He didn't even bother telling Linda about it.

But then, damned if Max didn't call two days later. He said he just wanted to let Lenny know he was working on Lenny's deal. "But I don't believe a thing until I see the first money," Lenny said. "So naturally, I figured I'd still keep my mouth shut."

Max called a few days later and offered Lenny the following deal. He, Max, would pay for Lenny and Linda to fly out there. He would find them a place to live, "nothing fancy, but you won't be ashamed." He would pay Lenny a thousand a week against a draw of one and a half percent of the gross sales Lenny rang up. And he would rent a car for Lenny.

By this time, Lenny was pretty excited. "You can work at this kind of thing your whole life and never even get close to getting a piece of the gross," Lenny said. "Usually, it's the net. Now I'm thinking I'm set for life. You can imagine. But still I play it very cool. I tell him that I'm thinking of a venture in Colorado that might be pretty good, too. And I tell him I'm thinking of going into the risk-arbitrage business. So he says that those businesses are shit compared with what I can make in L.A. That's when I tell him he's got to give me his prospect lists. And he says he will, and I tell him he's got a deal. We're leaving in three weeks."

I saw Lenny several times before he left. He was a changed person. Instead of the tales of persecution and woe, Lenny sang of deals and the man. He told me what he was going to have in Los Angeles: a Mercedes convertible; a black-bottomed swimming pool; a house with a view of the ocean; a sailboat; a cabin cruiser; a house in the desert; a ranch . . . I have forgotten the rest.

"There's no way they can stop me this time," Lenny said. "I have finally met a man who thinks big. This is a perfect partnership. He's got the deal and I can sell. It's perfect."

Linda was worried. She said they were already perfectly happy in New York. Besides, she didn't have any friends in Los Angeles. Lenny promised her that when you made a few million dollars, everyone was your friend.

Linda said she hoped she would be able to find a place to work where they would be as nice to her as they were at Murphy, Dunne, Dunne & Crutch. Lenny told her that there was no way on earth that she was going to work in Los Angeles. When a man reaches a certain level of income, his wife does not work. After all, Lenny had been telling Linda for years that she would not have to work for much longer. Now the day was at hand. Linda smiled, but she still looked worried. Unlike Lenny, Linda felt at home in her small world in Manhattan. She knew where she fit.

"I hope I can find a place where they teach ballet," Linda said. "Does anyone do ballet in California?"

Lenny said that he was going to spend every minute before he left boning up on the newest developments in tax laws. I never saw any tax books in his apartment. He did buy copies of *California Realités*, a magazine of estates and ranches in California, and *Palm Springs Life*. Linda bought three bottles of Sea'n'Ski suntan lotion.

Before Lenny left, he called a small synagogue in Coney Island. He told them he wanted to give away his furniture and appliances to a needy Russian Jewish immigrant. I was at their apartment the day before he left. The immigrant arrived, a thinner, more desperate version of Tevye the Dairyman. The immigrant stared at all the furniture, then pointed at the Panasonic TV and grunted. "No," Lenny said. "I'm taking that with me."

The immigrant looked disappointed, cheated. He sneered. Lenny said, "It's all right with me if you don't take any of it." The immigrant looked frightened and angry. With frantic sweeping movements he carried out a dining table, a queen-size bed, a chest of drawers, a bureau, a sideboard, four chairs, two reclining chairs, a convertible sofa, a chrome-and-foam-rubber modular sofa, and a matching chair. He stuffed it all into two elevators and then took it out to a car. It did not even take him an hour to empty Lenny's apartment, looking around all the time as if he might be stopped from carrying off these rich trophies of American life.

Lenny and Linda would get new furniture in Los Angeles. "It has to be very special furniture," Lenny said. "It has to be right for a southern California house. Really light and airy-looking. New York furniture wouldn't be right."

Linda nodded as if Lenny had said something brilliant.

Then they got into a taxicab and told the driver to take them to Kennedy Airport. Movers would come later for the hi-fi, the dishes, the pots, the Lichtenstein posters, the records, the Panasonic TV

Lenny had owned since college. Lenny had tipped the super twenty dollars to let the movers in. It was extravagant, but what was the point of having money if you didn't spend it?

The taxicab moved down York, then disappeared in morning traffic. I walked down toward Eighty-sixth in warm spring sunshine. I tried to think what lay ahead for Lenny. Linda had told me that she wished they were just subletting their apartment instead of giving it up. "What if we don't like it?" she asked me. "What if we want to move back here?"

Of course, Lenny would not have even thought the question was worth asking. Lenny did not doubt for a moment that if they ever came back to New York, they would stay in a suite at the Carlyle. Their old apartment would be suitable at most for their maid.

As for me, I knew I would miss Lenny a lot. In a way which I cannot articulate, I had become accustomed to his boasting, his self-deprecation, his plans, his scams. To me, they were a dialect which I had penetrated almost immediately. Behind the meaningless surface claims was an honesty about Lenny Brown which I rarely encountered in anyone else, if ever. Lenny said, over and over again, "Help me. I'm dying in a world I don't even belong in. Help me find my way home." Frankly, I thought that was what everyone would like to say. Lenny was just more honest in saying what was going on, which was another reason I liked him. I hoped that California would be home for him, a place for his soul to rest. And, in a way, that is what it was, but that was a long time off.

GOING FIRST-CLASS

Lenny Brown was no schmuck. Not by any means. Max Sherman knew it. That was why Max sent Lenny not just any tickets to Los Angeles, but first-class tickets. Lenny surprised Linda by showing her the tickets as they got to the airport. Not for them the endless lines of people boarding by row. They were all out of that mob with their SuperSaver ninety-nine-dollar fares; with their cheap clothes; their ratty carry-on bags; their torn wrappers around their Parisian bread; their children crying to go to the bathroom; their anxious, worried looks.

First-class means that the airline waits on you. You are doing them a favor to give them your custom. You are not hoping that the flight will be pleasant or that the chicken will be warm. There are people on the flight who are at your beck and call to make goddam sure that you are untroubled in every way that American Airlines can make possible.

Lenny and Linda had never flown first-class before. They had entered 707's and walked past the relaxed, bored-looking first-class passengers on their way to coach. It was embarrassing for all concerned, the passengers in first-class being obliged to hide behind their *Town & Country*'s while the cut-rate passengers tried to salvage a little dignity out of a hopeless situation. Lenny had always told Linda that someday they would travel first-class. They would sit two abreast, would have a wide choice of entrées, would relax and get some crucial work done. He had always told Linda it would happen, and now it was happening, right before their very eyes.

Even before the plane took off, the stewardess offered champagne or orange juice to Lenny and Linda. Lenny tried to act like he was bored by the whole thing, as if he had done it a hundred times before. He tried to act that way, but Linda saw right through it and started to giggle. Then Lenny started to giggle, too. A man with shaggy hair and a spreading waistline looked over at them from across the aisle. He nudged his traveling companion, a ravishing woman with a profile that was literally perfect. They smiled over at Lenny and Linda. Norman Mailer and Norris Church liked to see happy people.

When the seat-belt sign went off, the stewardesses set out a large tray of cheeses, sliced apples, pretzels, almonds, sausages, and Swedish meatballs in the middle of the first-class section. Lenny could see that the coach passengers got nothing. The stewardess politely asked the first-class passengers whether they preferred Rock Cornish game hen, prime rib, sea bass, fruit salad, or the kosher plate. Linda started to giggle again, but Lenny gave her a serious look and she stopped giggling.

Then the stewardess took drink orders. Lenny ordered a Chivas on the rocks. The stewardess brought it to him without batting an eye.

Linda ordered a split of Piper-Heidsieck champagne. She had seen ads for it in the *New Yorker*. The stewardess asked her if Moet & Chandon would be satisfactory.

Lenny got up and climbed the spiral staircase to the first-class lounge in the 747. He had never been in one before, although he had certainly seen pictures of them. He sat in a seat across from a love seat. Two women were sitting in the love seat. Both of them wore dresses that looked to Lenny as if they had come from one of those fancy stores on Madison Avenue. One of the women was middle-aged and almost preternaturally thin. She wore dark glasses inside the airplane. She was reading *The Fan Club*. On the third finger of her right hand she wore a square-cut emerald the size of a postage stamp. It covered her finger from the hand to the knuckle.

Lenny walked over to another table covered with food. He picked up a crab leg and started to eat it. He sat down next to the dish of crab legs. A thin man with wispy sideburns sat down on the other side of the crab legs. He ate one with dainty motions. Then he took out a thick book about the California budget for water conservation. Every few pages, Jerry Brown ate another crab leg.

Another man sat down next to Lenny on the other side. He was joined by an attractive young woman in skintight jeans and a T-shirt. Without a word, she took from a Hartmann leather attaché case a calculator with printing feature, a sheaf of spread sheets, and a piece of plain white paper. She started adding up the figures from a column in the spread sheets, then handed the piece of white paper with the totals to the man next to her.

He ran a hand through his straight brown hair and looked at his Peal loafers. His suit was immaculate, as if the tailor had just made it while the airplane was taxiing at Kennedy. "Do you mean to tell me that I am going to California for a syndicate that will net us no more than one point eight million?" he asked the girl. "I cannot believe that. Why couldn't our people in Los Angeles do it?"

"Company policy, John," the woman said. "A member of the board has to be there for everything over one point five."

"One point five is a small deal these days," the man said. "If only we had someone in L.A. who could add and subtract, we wouldn't have to waste my time on these rotten trips. I hate like hell to leave Sally up in Sharon all by herself for a deal like this. We've really got to find someone in L.A. we can trust."

"We've tried," the woman said. "There aren't that many good people in tax-shelter financing out there."

Lenny thought it would be disloyal to Max to talk to the man and woman. He filed away in his head, though, their need for someone who could handle exactly his specialty.

Lenny brushed by Jerry Brown on his way back to Linda. He felt light-headed from the emerald, the celebrities, the casual talk of one point eight million dollars.

"There's no doubt about it," Lenny said to Linda. "We're making the right move."

Linda grabbed Lenny's hand and squeezed it hard three times. A signal from their first days together at N.Y.U. *I love you.* Lenny squeezed Linda's hand four times. *I love you, too.* Tears of happiness flooded into Linda's blue eyes. She squeezed Lenny's hand twice.

How much? Lenny squeezed Linda's hand so hard that she winced. Then she kissed him. Norman Mailer made a gesture of applause. Linda thought that probably no one else on earth had ever been so happy.

"L.A. is a place where there's a lot of money floating around and very few people that Easterners can trust with it," Lenny said. "They have to send big executives out to L.A. when they could just have someone there all the time, if they trusted him. That's going to be me," Lenny said.

"That's probably exactly right," Linda said, looking at Lenny as if he had discovered relativity. "What kind of a place do you think they got for us? I hope it doesn't face an air shaft."

Lenny laughed out loud. "Max knows how important I am to his company," Lenny said. "Enough said. He wants to take very good care of me. That means getting us a decent place to live. I'm not worried about it."

For the next ten minutes, Lenny worried about it. Then their appetizers came. Baby bay shrimp, red Boston lettuce, another crab leg, salmon on a roll. Lenny had never known Linda to eat everything on her plate.

Lenny had another Chivas with his prime rib. Again, the stewardess did not hesitate for a moment. The Chivas slid down his throat clean and pure, with no aftertaste. The bargain scotches Linda bought at the Safeway almost always had an aftertaste. That was the taste of failure, the bitter sensation of spinning your wheels. Lenny thought he had finally left that feeling behind.

The stewardess asked the passengers to lower their window shades so that the movie could start. Then she passed out desserts— hot fudge sundaes with real fudge sauce heated up on a tray right in the aisle. There were also after-dinner drinks. The cabin grew dark as Lenny held a snifter of Courvoisier in his hand.

Of course, Lenny had eaten prime rib before, drunk Chivas before, tasted Courvoisier before. But those occasions were treats, made much of by all concerned. Now, in the first-class cabin, the stewardesses passed out *only* the best scotch, the tenderest meat, the most warming liqueurs. There was no fuss about it. It was assumed all around that you were accustomed to Chivas Regal. Luxury was a way of life for the first-class cabin.

Linda rested her head on Lenny's shoulder. She closed her eyes.

Lenny watched the movie for a few minutes, then turned the earphones to a classical channel. With a Mozart concerto for violins running through his head, Lenny drifted off into a drowsy trance.

In the first-class cabin, traveling forward to his destiny at six hundred miles per hour, a snifter of Courvoisier in his hand, sitting one seat behind the Governor of California, a stewardess eager to answer his any need, Lenny fell into a half-sleep of peace and happiness.

At last he was going to be the person he knew he could be.

TAKING OFF

Paint me a picture then. An Estes or a Goings. Photo-realist with the slick, glossy surfaces, the deceptively shallow depths, the hard edges, the aggressive confidence of two dimensions. Lenny and Linda in Los Angeles. A photo-realist portrait of a couple on the move.

Lenny hit the ground running. Max was waiting for him at the airport. In a Cadillac limousine with a bar, a television set, and a telephone. Max was a portly Jewish man in his fifties. He wore a cowboy suit and a silver belt buckle. He told Lenny it was a miracle that Lenny wound up with such a good-looking woman. "She's going to be popular in this town, boy," Max said. His stomach heaved with laughter. "You'd better make damned sure you keep an eye on her."

Linda blushed. Lenny felt embarrassed that he and Linda had such cheap luggage.

The limousine wended its way around the oval at LAX, then turned up Sepulveda Boulevard toward Westchester. Linda stared at the open, flat landscape. Hardly any of the buildings was more than two or three stories. In the distance there were mountains, but down near the airport, everything was flat. She could smell the sea air, even though she could not see the ocean.

The sunlight was dazzling. It was as if the sun were turned up twice as bright in Los Angeles, but without any more heat. New York had been far hotter. An almost cool overwhelming light, Linda thought.

There were no people on the streets. There were hardly any blacks. The cars all looked shiny and new. It was like a different world. Linda held her pocketbook. Inside were her typing test scores, just in case.

But what a ridiculous idea! Lenny and Max were already talking high finance. Max was telling Lenny about a project somewhere in West Los Angeles. Max was going to buy an old warehouse, refurbish it as offices, and rent it out. He needed investors to get together the down payment. The bank would lend them the rest of the money. There was a lot of talk about interest rates, points, depreciation, tax brackets—music to Lenny's ears.

"You just show me the guys who have the dollars," Lenny said. "That's all I want. I'll take over from there. Just let me have a crack at them."

Max Sherman laughed so hard that the limousine shook as they zoomed up La Cienega Boulevard. He clapped Lenny on the back. "That's my boy," he said. "That's the ticket. Don't be afraid to hustle. It's the ones who hustle who always get ahead. Always. No good worrying about getting your hands dirty. They get dirty if you don't hustle a lot faster than if you do. That's for sure."

"I'm not afraid to get my hands dirty," Lenny said.

Linda smiled at Max. "Lenny works really hard, Mr. Sherman," she said. "I've never known anyone who worked as hard as Lenny."

Lenny gave her a raised-eyebrow sign. He did not want her acting *too* eager to Max. She ought to have a little cool about her, as if she knew damned well that Lenny would be the best salesman Max ever had, and Max would find out for himself soon enough.

Soon the limousine rolled through West Hollywood, in front of the little Spanish row houses on Crescent Heights. "These are like gingerbread houses," Linda said.

"They start at a hundred twenty thousand," Max said. That was in 1976, and a hundred thousand for a house was a lot of money. Lenny did not act surprised, though. He had to keep his cool if he wanted Max to respect him. Linda just shook her head.

Then up to Sunset Boulevard. Linda and Lenny looked at the enormous billboards for rock performers he had never heard of.

Linda thought that billboards had been banned in most places. In Los Angeles, they were icons. Every other car was a Mercedes. Linda saw more Mercedes convertibles on the ride from the airport than she had seen before in her whole life. She wondered if they were cheaper in California. There were still no people on the sidewalks.

"My girl got you fixed up at a little place right up here," Max said. "I think it'll be all right. It's nothing fancy, but I don't think you'll have to be ashamed. I really don't." He chortled as he said it, as if he knew a secret.

Linda hoped it didn't look out on an air shaft. She had lived in a few places that did.

This one didn't. At the intersection of a steep hill called Kings Road and Hollywood Boulevard was a dream cottage with a sweeping view out over Los Angeles. It had a small front yard with a flagstone walk to the white front door. On both sides of the front door were rose bushes. Lenny and Linda could hardly believe their eyes. They stared like tourists.

"I think you'll like this," Max Sherman said, after he left them at the door with their luggage. "Call me tonight and I'll tell you where to meet me tomorrow."

Lenny felt like kissing Max's hands. He had only recently reached the stage of a one-bedroom apartment. Before that, they were all studios. Now he had a foyer, a dining room, a kitchen, a maid's room, a den, three bedrooms, and a deck that looked out over an enormous, throbbing city. The air was particularly clear on that first day. Lenny and Linda could see the beach at Marina del Rey. They could see the towers of downtown Los Angeles. They had no idea that the city was so enormous. There was low, densely built city as far as they could see. They were on the side of a mountain, overlooking it all.

They walked through the house like visitors to Versailles, looking at the Jenn-Air in the kitchen; the parquet hardwood floors in the living room; the bathtub fit for two in the "master suite," as Max had called it; the floor-to-ceiling windows in the living room; the built-in bookshelves in the den; and the dazzling sunlight flooding over everything, pouring in every window, bleaching out every doubt that they would live forever.

But the pool! Down a flight of stairs to a long, narrow playroom, bigger by itself than Lenny and Linda's apartment in New York, again the floor-to-ceiling windows, giving on the world's most perfect swimming pool. It was a rectangle with a jacuzzi built into one corner. Its waters were warmer than bathwater. It had a poolsweep. But far more than that, it had a black bottom, so that it did not look like a jerry-built afterthought in Levittown. Oh, no. This was the kind of pool that gets built by people who do *not* have to watch every penny. A black-bottomed pool, which Linda had read about in *Vogue*, was the exclusive prerogative of the rich. No installment buyers need apply.

Right then and there, without unpacking, Lenny took off his clothes and dove into the pool. Linda watched and giggled. Then she undressed and dove into the warm, clear waters. Why not? There were jacaranda trees everywhere, shielding Lenny and Linda from neighbors. This wasn't the suburbs, where someone's kid might walk in on them. This was where the stars lived, and stars valued their privacy and everybody else's. Lenny and Linda did surface dives, dive bombers, swam every which way, hugged and stroked each other in the warm waters of the jacuzzi. Everything else in their lives, they knew, had been a mere vale of tears before they got to this moment. This was what it meant to drink from the silver chalice.

But wait! The best was yet to come. There was a hallway leading from the downstairs gallery to a narrower hallway, which in turn led to a completely soundproofed, windowless room with acoustic tile on the walls and thick carpeting underfoot. Obviously a musician's lair. But how perfectly perfect! Probably the place had just been vacated by Rod Stewart or someone like that. What a great room for parties! What a great room just to sit in and be alone. No one could ever find them there.

It was warm in the room. Lenny and Linda were breathing hard from swimming. They were naked. They made love right there on the thick, soundproof rug. Then they lay on their backs and looked at the ceiling.

"I hope it never ends," Linda said.

"It's just beginning," Lenny said. "Someday this place will be just the kind of place for our servants. We'll be in a much bigger place, and we'll come to this place and just remember when we were starting out."

"No," Linda said, "this is enough. This is all I ever wanted."

"Think big," Lenny said. "Think big."

And even that was not the end. When Lenny was looking for a place to stash their suitcases, he came upon a door which led to a darkened garage. He fumbled for a light switch. When he flipped on the light, there, sitting in the garage like the earthly incarnation of divinity, was a gleaming tobacco-brown Mercedes convertible, a 450 SL with the Keys in the ignition and a note on the leather driver's seat. "It never hurts to make a good impression," said the note, with Max's flamboyant signature.

If Max Sherman had been Satan, if he had torn out Lenny's fingernails, he could not have motivated Lenny any more. Lenny had been taken up to the top of the mountain, shown all the kingdoms of the west side of Los Angeles, and now was ready to do Max's bidding, whatever it was.

To tell the truth, it wasn't even painful. Lenny liked to sell. It was an outlet for his overpowering aggressiveness, a way to impose his will on others and, in return, get their money so as to buy for Linda and for himself all the things they deserved.

The very first day on the job, Max met Lenny at Max's office in Century City. The offices were on the fortieth floor of a building facing west. From Lenny's very own office, the first office of his own he had ever had, Lenny could see far out to sea. The ocean sparkled and glittered all the way back to him in his office. He could see the surf breaking in a white line all the way up the coast.

Max sketched out the details of the first project Lenny would work on, the warehouse-conversion project near Santa Monica. It was a fairly straightforward deal. All Lenny had to do was persuade a few dentists who had some income to shelter that this project would be the perfect deal. "I want you to lean very heavily on the fact that you're from New York," Max said. "That carries a lot of weight with people here."

Lenny and Max met the two dentists together, which Lenny also liked a lot. In New York, he had always been sent out by himself. He thought it showed a good spirit, a real desire to work together, lots of confidence in the future, for Max to come along. Drs. Weinglass and Shapiro pulled up in a gray Porsche at the warehouse site. They were short little men in jogging suits. They both squinted from wearing contact lenses.

Lenny had done a lot of selling. He was looking for fifty thou each from the dentists. He knew that people do not part with that kind of money easily. It took a helluva sell.

Wrong, Lenny, wrong. In L.A., people will buy anything! The doctors were signing the papers after a half hour. No crap about reading the fine print, no bullshit about having their lawyers go over everything with a fine-tooth comb. Lenny laid out the deal, told them that the appreciation possibilities were better in that area than anywhere else in America, that—based on his long New York experience—the IRS could not possibly question the deductions, answered a few questions about who would pay for extraordinary repairs—and that was it!

"The thing is," Dr. Weinglass said with a smile, "it's a lot better than throwing the money down a rathole for my wife's brother, which is what'll happen to it if I don't put it somewhere she can't get at it."

Shapiro simply said that he had to attend a seminar on private financing of motion pictures so that he had to get going. "I'm sorry," he said. "We'll talk more some other time."

In less than an hour, Lenny was back at the office, calculating that he had made about fifteen hundred dollars the first hour he had worked.

Max took Lenny into his corner office—triangular, in fact, since the building was a triangle—and gave him a Johnny Walker Black. Then he told Lenny to sit down on his glove-leather tan and chrome couch. Max patted his stomach as if he had eaten a good meal and said, "Lenny, you are going to go very far in this town. I don't know if you realize just how good you are. There's a sincere quality about you, a concerned quality, as if you really cared about whether people did well on their investments. It's not just hype to you. You care for people. In our business, that's the bottom line. Caring for people."

Max did have a few pointers. Lenny should definitely not promise people that the IRS would not disallow the shelter. After all, the IRS was crazy. They might do anything. Another thing was to avoid being quite so specific on the points that were not covered in the large type of the prospectus. "Sometimes it's in the investor's best interest not to be scared out of a really advantageous deal by a few scare words in the fine print."

Finally, the dentists were the perfect investors. They had obviously been cheating like hell on their income taxes and needed some way to cover up. "If a guy looks like he's really serious about finding a tax shelter that would stand up under an electron microscope, we probably don't want him. Once they start whining about their lawyers, just forget about them."

Lenny knew the score. "Lawyers are deal breakers," he said back to Max. "Salesmen are deal makers. That's the whole difference."

Max slapped Lenny on the back. "That's it exactly. You're here because you can sell," he said. "I have two lawyers from Harvard Law School. Or maybe Yale. I bring them with me into the toilet when I shit. If I get tired of them, I get two others. They're a dime a dozen. Guys like you are rare."

Lenny had been working in sales for a lot of years. This was the first time anyone had ever spoken to him like that, as if he were really somebody worth talking to, somebody you'd be proud to have around. Lenny looked out the window. He felt as if he could fly.

Max and Lenny talked for a while, and Lenny told Max for the tenth time how grateful he was for the house and the car. "Listen, pal," Max said, "you're going to earn those things. I would never have gotten them for you if I hadn't known for a fact that you were going to make me even richer than I am now."

"You can put the money in the bank," Lenny said. "You can spend it."

"Damn," Max said. "I like that. I don't think you even really know just how good you are."

If you take a man who has always gotten by on self-promotion, self-encouragement, self-starting in his work, and if you then show that man how to make fifteen hundred dollars in an hour, shower him with praise, and tell him he is better than he realizes, you are going to have a man who is delirious with joy. That was Lenny after his first day of work.

He drove home in the afternoon breeze of Los Angeles. He pulled up to other Mercedes convertibles at stoplights. He gave the drivers knowing looks. "I know how it's done," he said by those looks. "I know just as well as you how to get money. I'm in the club."

At the corner of Santa Monica Boulevard and Doheny, Lenny stopped at a florist. Lenny bought a dozen long-stemmed roses for Linda. He did not have any cash, so he put the charge on his American Express card.

Linda had been home all day. She had unpacked all their clothes. She had ironed some of them. She dusted all the bookshelves and the dining table. Then she vacuum-cleaned the carpet in the study. She found a rake and brushed away a few leaves in the front yard. A neighbor passed by walking an Afghan hound, but the neighbor did not talk to Linda. Linda used a broom to sweep up around the black-bottomed pool. There was really nothing to sweep up, but Linda wanted to do something useful, so that Lenny would know that she was keeping up her end.

In one of the closets, Linda found a stack of BankAmericard bills for a previous tenant of the house. They were for immense sums for meals at restaurants with French names. Linda was embarrassed to read them, but she did, anyway. After all, the man had left them there. Month by month, in 1974, the tenant had accumulated a larger bill, until one final bill appeared notifying him that his credit limit was passed, and since no payments had been received for the last several months, his credit card had to be returned. BankAmericard asked that the card be cut in two and sent back in the enclosed envelope. The enclosed envelope was still enclosed. Linda threw out all the bills. They gave her the creeps.

She thought of walking down the hill to a grocery store, but she did not know how far away the closest one might be. Plus, she might get lost and have to call Lenny at work. Above all, she did not want to disturb him at work.

She rummaged through her belongings and found her typing scores, her shorthand record, and a "To whom it may concern" letter of recommendation from Mrs. O'Leary, the office manager at Murphy, Dunne, Dunne & Krutch. She read the letter. Mrs. O'Leary said that Linda was a reliable worker whom they were sorry to lose, who could be counted on to give 100 percent for whomever employed her.

Lenny had told her that she did not have to get a job, that she would never have to get a job again, but Linda thought it was better to be safe than sorry. If things did not work out as well as Lenny hoped, she wanted to be ready to pitch in.

There was a Los Angeles telephone directory in the kitchen. Linda looked up dance studios. She called a few of them. She found one in Hollywood which sounded good. It was inexpensive, only five dollars per lesson, and the teacher sounded serious about the dance. If she and Lenny could afford to get another car, she would arrange to take lessons. Unless Lenny thought it was too extravagant. After all, when you moved to a new town, you had a lot of expenses getting started. Maybe she would put off mentioning ballet to Lenny until they had a chance to sort out how much money they were going to have. There had just been too many times when Lenny had said they were all set when they were not all set at all, when there had been a boss who didn't think big enough or who didn't appreciate how a *really* good salesman sold.

There was no sense in rushing things. Who could tell? They might wind up going back to New York in a few months. Lenny was a brilliant man, but sometimes he had trouble getting along with the people he worked for.

Linda read her guidebook about places to eat in Hollywood for five dollars or less. She still had two hours before Lenny would get home, so she changed into her red one-piece bathing suit and went down to the pool. She had a small portable radio, which she played as she lay on a towel on an aluminum and plastic beach chair. The disk jockey on the radio interrupted the program every fifteen minutes to give the surf report. "This is Woody Kling in Laguna. Waves are four to five feet, and shape is fair to good," went a typical report.

It was only four-thirty in the afternoon. To think that a few days before, she would have been at work, getting ready to take a subway, and now she was lying by her own swimming pool on a brilliant, sunshiny day, listening to music and surf reports! Even if it did not last, she would remember this day for as long as she lived. The luxury of lying by your own pool, all by yourself, without screaming children around like at the pool club she used to go to when she was a child, well, it was pretty wonderful that Lenny had gotten them to this stage.

She was changed and made up when Lenny got home. He handed her the roses and kissed her. She had never seen him smiling like that. He hugged her and kissed her again.

"This has been the best day of my life," he said.

Linda wanted to make dinner at home, to save a few dollars, but Lenny insisted on taking her out. Linda told him restaurants for five dollars a person and less while Lenny told her about his day. When he got to the part about Max saying that even he didn't know how good he was, Linda started to cry with happiness. To see her Lenny, who had been treated so meanly by so many people, treated at last with the kind of respect he deserved was like a gift from heaven.

Lenny was not about to take her out to some five-dollar-and-under restaurant. He had heard people at the office talking about a French place called Ma Maison. He guessed it was expensive, but he didn't care. What was the point of having a gift for making money if you didn't enjoy it? Linda thought it was extravagant, but she did not want to spoil Lenny's fun.

Ma Maison was only a few minutes from their house. It was basically just a small house with a few tables inside and then a covered-over parking lot paved with astro-turf. The maitre d' was a little snobby, but the food was wonderful.

"This is just the beginning," Lenny said every few minutes. "There's no way that anybody's going to stop me now. I always knew this kind of job was out there. Now it's going to be Katie, Bar The Door."

Linda could not believe how well things were going. The food came in tiny portions, but Linda was too excited to eat, anyway. Lenny had figured out that if he made fifteen hundred dollars each day he worked, he would make about three hundred seventy-five thousand a year. Linda's head swam. "But it'll actually be much more than that," Lenny said. "Max told me that he would give me bigger and bigger deals to handle as I learned the ropes and stuff."

Across the room, at a table close to the door, Jerry Brown was eating dinner with a paunchy man with a bald head. Lenny thought he should go over and remind the Governor that they had all flown out on the same flight. Linda said that might embarrass him. "Anyway," she said, "it just proves that we'll be seeing a lot more of him, so we can do it another time."

Lenny ordered a bottle of Moet & Chandon champagne without asking how much it cost. "If you have to ask how much everything costs," he said, "where's the fun of making money? Really," he added, "we deserve it."

The bottle of champagne cost forty-eight dollars. Lenny acted as if it did not matter, but Linda could see that he was surprised.

At home, Linda asked Lenny how she would get around. "If I knew where on this street to catch the bus, I could take a bus," she said. "But I don't see any signs of a bus stop anywhere."

"There aren't any buses up here," Lenny said. "I don't know that there are any buses anywhere in this whole town. Anyway, are you kidding? You think I would have my wife take a bus? This weekend we're going to go out and get you a car. You've got to have a car."

"Really, Lenny?" Linda asked. She had never owned her own car. Not ever.

"What kind of a car would you like?" Lenny asked. "If I can have a nice car, you can have a nice car, too. That's only fair."

"Anything would be fine," Linda said. "Maybe a Pinto. They're supposed to get great mileage."

Lenny smiled and chucked Linda's chin. He already knew what kind of car she wanted. She had once pointed one out in a James Bond movie, back in the days when it was just a joke to her, back in the days before Lenny came into his own.

They stopped at the liquor store at La Cienega and Sunset to buy a bottle of Amaretto. They swam naked in their pool, drank Amaretto as they sat in the jacuzzi, and then they slept an innocent sleep.

For the next month, Lenny was a house afire. He worked every day, including Sundays. He sold out that warehouse renovation before the end of the month. The dentists and doctors and lawyers and airline pilots came in and out, and Lenny explained to all of them why the property was certain to go up in value far beyond what they had dreamed of. Lenny explained the tax write-offs. He never promised anyone that the scheme would not be audited, or gave any guarantees that it would hold up in tax court. The questions simply never came up because Lenny was so goddam good that, after he had finished laying it on about the top tax firm which had drawn up the deal, the former judge of the Federal tax court who had given his seal of approval, the going over by Home Savings & Loan's legal department, the topflight people from every walk of life who had already invested in the project—stars, corporate tycoons, sports figures with hawk-eyed business managers—after all that, the investors would have been too embarrassed even to question the deal. It was not only the facts and figures, but the quality of human caring that Lenny put into each and every contact. Lenny would think long and hard before parting with fifty or a hundred thousand or a quarter of a million of his dollars, and the clients should do the same.

But for every client, Lenny had the perfect answer to why the papers should be signed right then and there. The deal was almost closed out. The federal tax regs were about to be altered so that a deal like this would be just a sweet memory if you got in, a bitter taste if you didn't. If you signed up right away, there was a good possibility that you would get money back from rents in the first year. People who signed up next month would have to wait until calendar 1978 at the earliest. People who signed up now would be wrapped under the syndicator's employer's I.D. number so that their investments would be just between them, the IRS, and Lenny. No one, not even wives or children, would have to know about it. If you signed up right away, Lenny and Max would certainly consider you for their next project, which was approximately the equivalent of buying land in Beverly Hills in 1976 at 1950 prices.

The cardboard-box manufacturers and chiropodists and car dealers and real-estate brokers came and went. They almost always left their signed participations in the deal. Their checks invariably followed right away.

Even if they did not buy in, they went away liking Lenny because he was a sincere guy. If you didn't buy, he would simply shake your hand, tell you he appreciated the opportunity of talking with you, and that would be the end of it. No snide comments. Just a warm handshake and the feeling that Lenny Brown cared about people.

The deals these textile manufacturers, dress designers, medical-supply salesmen and engineers came away with were good deals. They would lower tax liability by far more than they cost. If the real-estate market continued to boom, they would make a capital gain on their initial investment, too.

For Max Sherman and Co., d/b/a Century West Equities, the deals were even sweeter. First of all, right off the top, there was a 4 percent sales fee. That money was gone into Max and Lenny's pockets to buy meals at Ma Maison and lease Mercedes convertibles. Then, Century West Equities owned twenty percent of the project for the effort and risk of being the general partner. If the investors put in five million, if the mortgage were twenty million, then Century West Equities immediately owned as much as all the other investors put together.

That was sweet, but what was even sweeter was that the general partner got the first profits out in case of sale up to six million dollars. If that was all the profit there was, too bad for the dentists, cardboard-box manufacturers, and airline pilots.

Then the building would need a management company, which got a large percentage of the rents. The management company's function was to provide "management advice," which is to say that it did nothing. Then there was a yearly fee out of the rents for keeping the air-conditioning running, disinfecting the men's room, and otherwise making certain that the building stayed in topflight condition. That function was performed by Century West Building Maintenance and Supply, a subsidiary of Century West Equities.

By the time the project was fully bought, Max Sherman could look forward to a lifetime of financial security. Why would the investors give such a staggering gift to Uncle Max? Because they did not care about Max Sherman. They cared only that because of every fifty thousand they put into the project, they got to deduct two hundred thousand from their taxable income. For those in the fifty percent bracket, that meant two dollars back right off the top for every dollar they put in. Plus the possibility of a capital gain. Max's project had a good reputation for paying off on the capital-gains side.

The investors were unconcerned that the poor fool working for a weekly paycheck, getting money taken out on withholding, would have to make up the difference. In this world, as Lenny said, if you have arms, you take. People with the kind of money which needs tax shelters know the lesson well.

And anyway, who cares about all this social crap? The way the world works is that if you fall into something lucky, you don't start whining about social justice. You get what you can, and that's that. Lenny did not even think about it for one second. He had sold half of the renovated warehouse; he was down for $37,500—before taxes—in the first month he was in L.A.

It was more than he had ever earned in any three years of his life before.

Lenny was a pistol, glowing red-hot in the southern California night. He could do no wrong. As far as he was concerned, he was immortal. Every few days I would get a deliriously happy phone call from Lenny. "It's so good," he would say. "It's exactly the way I always hoped it would be. This is a place where you can make anything you want out of yourself. Out here, everything is the way it's supposed to be."

Lenny called me one day while I was at my desk at the *Wall Street Journal*. The man behind me screamed with laughter because the Secretary of the Treasury had told New York City to go bankrupt

GARDNER-WEBB COLLEGE LIBRARY
P. O. Box 836
Boiling Springs, N.C. 28017

and be damned. From across the continent, Lenny told me how he had surprised his wife with a white Jaguar coupé. He had given it to her right outside their house in the Hollywood Hills, just after they had gotten out of the pool. He told me that when I was soaked to the bone from walking across Cortlandt Street back from lunch at a Greek hamburger stand in a rainstorm. "It's great out here," Lenny said. "When are we going to see you?"

From my gray metal desk at the *Wall Street Journal*, I envied Lenny's optimism, his joy. I told him I would see him in a week. The *Journal* was sending me out to cover a convention of the National Association of Broadcasters in Las Vegas. I could use my own money to go on to L.A.

"Once you see how it is here," Lenny said, "you won't want to come back."

He was right. Lenny met me at the airport in a limousine with a television in the back seat. I had never been in a car like that. He had champagne in an icebox in the back seat. We drank and watched "General Hospital" as the car took me up to the Beverly Hills Hotel. Lenny had wanted me to stay with him, but I wanted to be certain that I was not a burden, a legacy of thought from Mom.

He and Linda took me to dinner at Ma Maison. By then, he knew the maitre d', Patrick. He was sitting much closer to the front door than he had when he first came. "That's what comes of putting a few twenties in his hand," Lenny said. "When I first came here, I didn't know what the difference between a good table and a bad table even was."

Linda was smiling, healthy-looking, full of stories of the people in her ballet class. "A woman in my class told me she was absolutely convinced that she was the reincarnation of Henry Wadsworth Longfellow's wife. She was dead serious. She told me she was going to Boston to read his diaries just to make sure her dreams weren't lying." Linda told me that story while the waiter asked M'sieur Brown if he would like his usual wine, the Puligny-Montrachet.

"Where are the little places where the owner has to know you to let you in?" I asked. "The places nobody knows about but you?"

Lenny laughed and said, "That's where we're going tomorrow night. To a little Italian place where the owner is a friend. He hasn't had any new customers in two years, but I did him a favor with some people who had loaned him money."

Linda winked at me and said, "And now the guy is Lenny's slave for life."

Lenny caught the wink, squeezed Linda's hand, and winked back. I was impressed. Only a couple who are confident about themselves and their place in the world around them can afford to be self-aware.

When the salad came, Lenny ate it with the dinner fork. Linda noticed but said nothing. It would be insane to criticize the dinner manners of a man who has made over $37,500 in his first month in town.

"Of course, I don't just get a check for that amount," Lenny said. "There are a lot of expenses that I have to pay, and since I get a share of the gross, Max says I should pay for part of the overhead. That's only fair. After all, if there were no overhead there, how would I get anything sold?"

After everything, though, Lenny had made twenty thousand in that first month. To me, who made four hundred thirty dollars a week, Lenny might as well have been making a billion dollars a day.

Lenny had two new toys he wanted to show me. In his study, he had three television sets in a blond wood console right next to each other, with a remote-control device next to a large black leather easy chair. "This is really important," Lenny said. "I can use this to keep up on fast-breaking news stories. LBJ had one just like it. I can keep the sound up on one and then turn down the sound on it and turn up the sound on another one if it looks like there's something important happening on the other network."

"Is this for business?" I asked.

"Absolutely," he said. "Anything that affects the economy or interest rates or taxes can be crucial in my business."

"I'm amazed he got along for so long without it," Linda said. They both laughed, and Lenny hugged Linda. Again, these were signs of a couple on the move. To me, they were far more important signals than a good table at Ma Maison or a Mercedes convertible.

Lenny still had his Panasonic that he had owned all through college. Linda said, "I don't think he'll ever get rid of that."

In the living room, overlooking the lights of the city, Lenny had a new brass telescope. It was mounted on a tripod and looked as if it worked.

"I use this to remind myself that there are other people up at night," Lenny said. "With this, I can see people's lights going on and off in their houses."

I had to interview a famous television producer the next day, but I met Linda for lunch. "It's really true," she said while she ate a tiny salad at a horrible place called The Moustache Cafe. "I have never seen Lenny like this. It's like he was a rosebush that had all these beautiful flowers in it, but nobody had ever watered it. And now flowers are coming out all over it."

"But Linda," I said, "you watered it. You've been devoted to him for an awfully long time."

"I know," she said. "But a man in this world needs more than somebody who cares about him. He needs to feel that he's just as good as other men. That's what it's all about to Lenny. He needs to feel as if he's going to be rich, to have people respect him. That's what counts for Lenny."

I looked around that restaurant. It seemed to me to be only a tent erected on top of a parking lot which was then covered over with astro-turf. At every table were men who looked as if they had seen every trick in the book and had thought of a few new ones to wring a dollar out of an unyielding earth. The women, in their jogging outfits and their fuck-me pumps, looked even more crazed and dangerous than the men. Los Angeles is the only place I have ever been where the women look harder and more desperate than the men. In the midst of these piranhas sat Linda. She was a person of shocking kindness, a throwback to a different era. I wondered how long Lenny would last in that swamp without Linda to throw him a rope every day.

Linda could tell what I was thinking. "I know the people in L.A. are weird-looking," she said. "But Lenny really gets along well with them. He really has a good sense of what they like and how to get them to buy things from him."

"Does he have any friends?" I asked.

"Oh, absolutely," Linda said. "He has this great friend named Joel who really likes him." Linda bobbed her head enthusiastically. "Joel's made millions out of the car-wash business. He and Lenny spend a lot of time talking about real estate."

"Do you have friends?" I asked. "People you can talk to about something other than real estate?"

"Oh, yes," Linda said. "I have a wonderful friend who works as a secretary at some law firm. Just like I did in New York before we came out here. She's really funny. She's in point class just like me. She thinks there are people among us who came here from other planets. That's what she told me. But she's not the same one who thinks she's Henry Wadsworth Longfellow's wife."

Linda drove me around Hollywood in a rented car. It was a strange place, with low, abandoned hamburger stands next to expensive decorators. Then she drove me to Beverly Hills. She wanted to show me how much the houses cost. We drove by large colonial houses situated a few feet from the next house. There were magnificent royal palms all along the street. Every car had a Rolls-Royce parked in front. She pointed at a particularly well-kept house on Roxbury Drive.

"That's Joel's house," Linda said. "He paid two hundred fifty thousand for it. Now it's worth a million and a half. That's what he told Lenny. Lenny thinks it's worth even more."

"Amazing," I said. It looked like an ordinary house, but a house which makes its owner a millionaire is no ordinary house.

"Joel bought that house when he was twenty-seven years old. He had already made two million cash by then. From buying and selling car washes," Linda said. "He told Lenny that Lenny would be richer than he was by a long way."

"Did Lenny like that?" I asked.

Abruptly Linda looked sad. "Yes," she said. "He liked it a lot."

"But he wondered why he wasn't richer already, right?" I asked.

"Exactly," she said.

I had to think of Lenny, a man who thought that the only thing in life that counted was how much money you bring home, in the company of a Joel, who had already brought home so much money. When I thought of that, it reminded me of a man who is told that no matter what he does, he will always have a crippling pain in his side. Nothing will be able to take it away. To put a man as competitive as Lenny into a world in which there were million-and-a-half dollar houses a few feet apart for miles on end was like putting a wolf into a trap. The wolf would be bound either to die or chew off its leg to get free. That was how it seemed to me at the time, but I am a notoriously bad judge of character. In addition, I knew little of Los

Angeles. I could easily have misjudged it completely. At least no one was laughing hysterically about quarter-point changes in the depreciation allowance.

I asked Linda if we could see the Los Angeles County Art Museum. "It's not worth seeing," she said. "I've been there. It's empty."

Linda had a good eye, so I took her word for it. Los Angeles is an interesting town. When you visit, the residents want to show you the expensive stores and restaurants and fabulously expensive homes, and these are impressive, just as it would be impressive to visit Fort Knox. But there is nothing beautiful to see. No museums, no parks, no art galleries. The only things worth seeing are the artifacts of how much money is to be made there. Los Angeles proclaims proudly that in the pursuit of money, all other concerns have been jettisoned.

That night, Linda and Lenny took me to a party at Joel's house on Roxbury Drive. Lenny was tired from a day of selling participations in a South Bay shopping center to a group of Iranian chewing-gum magnates, but he insisted on going to the party, anyway.

"Joel has a party almost every night," Lenny said. "Linda and I like to go when we have nowhere else to go. It's usually a lot of fun. He likes me. He's like taking me under his wing."

We drove over to the party. There were two female valets parking the cars. There were only Porsches, Mercedes convertibles, and Rolls-Royces at the party. No other kinds of cars.

A Mexican maid greeted us at the front door. She knew Lenny and Linda, which was the occasion for obvious pride on Lenny's part. "How are you, Mistuh Brow'?" she asked.

"Just fine, Elena," Lenny said.

There was disco music coming from the living room. But there was no one in the living room. Instead, there was a stereo even more elaborate than Lenny's playing music while computerlike lights flashed on it. The living room was furnished entirely in white. White walls, white sofas, white love seats, white shag rugs, even white paintings in white plastic frames. The only color was from the stereo.

There were even white sculptures of women's torsos, complete with etchings of pubic and underarm hair on the white stone.

A row of white French doors gave onto the most beautiful swimming pool and backyard I had ever seen. The pool was large, rectangular, lit by many small lights running around the sides of the pool underwater. It was surrounded by decking and then a lawn which looked like the ninth green at Pebble Beach. There were chairs and lounges. There was a long table of food. Several servants in black livery circulated around the pool area passing out drinks and snacks. There were about twenty people lying around the pool. Only one woman, a girl with a maillot cut about up to her neck, swam lazily back and forth in the pool.

I walked out to the pool with Lenny and Linda. The guests were gathered in small knots talking to each other. They looked at us as we came in but said nothing to us until we had reached the brick decking. Then several of them greeted Lenny and Linda. They then turned back to their conversations.

The men were almost all young, slightly overweight, bearded, wearing trousers that were too tight for them, thin leather jackets, and, yes, little necklaces. Almost all of the men were squinting, which meant that they were still adjusting to wearing contact lenses. The women were all thin. They wore tight jeans and T-shirts. Most of them wore medium-height backless pumps, fuck-me pumps. The women did not look as if they were listening to any of the conversation. They seemed to be off in their own worlds somewhere. While the men talked about deals and taxes, the women studied their fingernails. Every woman there had beautiful nails. The women were generally extremely attractive in a cheap way, which is not meant as a criticism at all. It means only that the women apparently believed they were there to display their bodies and their faces, which they did as effectively as the *Wall Street Journal* pushed supply-side economics.

Lenny guided us over to a short, painfully thin man (the only one there) with a gray beard and a youthful face. The man wore wire-rimmed glasses. His teeth were crooked. To me, he looked like a Yeshiva *bucher* with Gucci shoes, an open-necked Hermes shirt, and gold chains. He smiled at Lenny as if he had just noticed that we had arrived. He put his arm around Lenny and squeezed Lenny's shoulders. "How's the hottest thing in Los Angeles?" he asked. "How's the boy who's going to make all of us look like welfare mothers?"

Lenny actually blushed. "Joel," Lenny said, "I'd like you to meet my friend Ben. He writes columns for the *Wall Street Journal*. Joel Miller, this is Ben Stein."

Lenny smiled at me cheerfully as if he had just caught a prize marlin, which he could then show off to his friends. Joel looked at me seriously. "I love the *Wall Street Journal*," he said. "It's the only newspaper I allow in my house. As far as I'm concerned, it's the only one that's honest."

We talked for a few minutes about the *Wall Street Journal*. It took some time for me to impress upon Joel that I wrote far more about "Laverne and Shirley" than about real-estate investment trusts, but Joel did not care. "In this town, people will be all over you when they hear you're with the *Wall Street Journal*," he said. "You might write something about them that would make money for them."

"I doubt it," I said. Lenny looked embarrassed, so I added, "Of course, I'm always looking for new stories."

Joel shuffled off to talk to someone who had just come in. I stood with Lenny and Linda. We were an island of strangers at a party of people who knew each other's income-tax returns. Lenny did not know any of the other guests, as far as I could tell. Linda smiled as if she were glad to be there.

A woman in a T-shirt and jeans came over to talk to Linda. They had been in the same dance class. A man came over to talk to Lenny. Joel had sent him to ask Lenny about getting in on the ground floor on some tax-shelter scheme in Riverside County. The man put his arm around Lenny and led him off to a dark corner of the pool grounds, as if an agent of the IRS might overhear their conversation.

I stood in the light of a spotlight, eating a *rumaki*. A black-haired woman with dark blue eyes came over to me. "Joel says you're from the *Wall Street Journal*," she said.

"That's right," I said.

"Does that pay much?" she asked.

"No," I said.

"I figured that," she said. "That's a fucked way to live. Having to depend on people like Joel for your money."

"I don't know what you mean," I said.

"Half the people here are getting their rent paid by the other half," she said. "Guess which half is which."

When the woman moved her face out of the shadow of the spotlight, I could see that she was genuinely beautiful. She had perfect lips and a small, little girl's nose. "Joel tells me that your pal Lenny is making a lot of money," she said.

"I think he is," I said.

"He'd better be," she said. "His name is Joe Shit if he doesn't make some real money in this crowd. Joel used to have this friend who was really, really big in T-shirt transfers. He had this factory out near the airport. He was grossing seven or eight million a year. He and Joel were like brothers. They couldn't see enough of each other. I used to see him here every night. Joel told me he liked the guy so much that he wouldn't mind if I fucked him. That's how much he liked him. Then the guy lost the franchise on the transfers, which is handled by some very nice people in Cleveland, and the schmuck is out of work in five minutes and his factory is gone and the guy is a salesman for some stationery company now. He sells office supplies over the phone. You think Joel returns his calls? You're crazy if you do."

Linda had overheard this conversation. The corners of her mouth looked pinched and anxious. "I think Joel likes Lenny just because they have a lot of fun together," Linda said.

The woman smiled as one might smile at a retarded child. "You think so?" she asked. "You think anyone in this town likes anyone else who doesn't make money? You think there's anything in this whole town except people looking for what somebody else can do for them?"

"The women in my dance class don't expect anything from me," Linda said.

"Oh, yes. The women in your dance class. That means a helluva lot," said the woman with the perfect nose. "That means a great, great deal," she said, shaking her head. Then she walked away.

Later, as I was coming out of the bathroom of Joel's pool house, Joel put his arm around me. "Your friend is very, very hot," he said. "Very hot."

"That's great," I said. "He deserves it."

Another man came over. He was plump, short, with peering brown eyes. He wore a beard. Joel introduced him as Michael. Joel said that Michael was "very possibly the largest factor in automobile detailing kits" in Los Angeles. A "detailing kit" is an elaborate set of detergents and waxes for making your car look like new. Joel told Michael that I worked for the *Wall Street Journal*. Michael said that the *Journal* had not yet done a piece on the detailing business, "which is really one of the key businesses in California," as he said.

While we talked about detailing, a woman in white jeans and a black T-shirt walked by. Her bosoms were miraculous.

"I'd like to get into that," Michael said.

"I wouldn't call it the impossible dream," Joel said. "You've got all the 'ludes in the world."

Michael raised his eyebrows and said, "We'll see."

Joel and Michael said they would see me later and walked away. Lenny came over. "I think I've just made a very major sale," he said. "Wait till I tell Max Sherman about this. That guy is taking five or six thousand a week out of a couple of adult bookstores in Sherman Oaks. He needs a place to park it for a while."

Linda smiled at Lenny. "I'm a little tired," she said. "Can we go home?"

"In just a few minutes," Lenny said. "That guy is talking to another friend of his. He's going to see if he can buy the whole project just between the two of them. Then we might not have to report it to the IRS." He took Linda's hand. "It'll just take a few minutes."

Linda and I went into the living room. We sat down on a white couch. The woman with the perfect nose sat on the white couch across from our white couch. She looked at us with her dark blue eyes. The pupils were as big as Frisbees.

"Sometimes I get so fucking sick of Joel and his low-life friends that I wish I could just get on a plane and take off and never come back," she said without preamble.

Linda and I smiled at her. Linda said that she was sorry that the woman was so upset. "Joel's really a pretty nice guy when you get to know him," Linda said.

"You think I don't know him?" she said. "I know him plenty. Too much." She shook her head derisively. "I know him enough to know that he still calls his mother every day to tell her if his shit is coming out all right or if he's constipated or has diarrhea. You think I don't know him?"

Lenny appeared at the French doors. He looked at me, looked at Linda, then looked at the girl with the perfect nose. "Hi, Rochelle," he said. "Linda and Ben, this is Rochelle. She's living with Joel."

Rochelle sat up bolt upright on the couch. "I'm not living with Joel," she corrected. "I am a stewardess for United Airlines. I sometimes stay here when I'm in town," she said, "but I do not live here. Did Joel tell you I live here?" she demanded.

"Take it easy, Rochelle," Lenny said. "You know Joel never says anything bad about you."

"You think I have to depend on people like Joel?" Rochelle asked. "Listen, pal," she said, "I've been on airplanes with people who took me out to dinner and then I let them take me back to their hotels and then the next morning they took me to Tiffany and told me to just pick out anything I wanted. Anything at all. You think Joel's ever done that?"

"I think we'd better go now," I said.

"Listen, Lenny, you cute little guy who thinks that Joel's so great, I could tell you things about how Joel can't sleep for a week if he doesn't get a letter from his mother. You think he's so great because he made a lot of money in car washes? You think that's great? He's so fucking scared that he's going to lose it that he stays up all night adding things up on his calculator," Rochelle said. She shook her head in a gesture of anger at herself. "Listen, pal," she said to the floor, "there are still guys in this country who can't sleep thinking about what I did to them the first night I met them. I still get letters from guys I spent one night with five years ago. And I'm spending my time with Joel Miller? Who thinks he's a sport because he owns a few car washes?" She shook her head in disbelief.

I looked up at the French doors. Joel stood there with a tight little smile on his face. "I think you ought to let Ben and Lenny and Linda go home now, Rochelle," he said. "I'll bet they're really tired."

Rochelle did not lift her eyes from the floor. Very distinctly, under her breath, she said, "You little faggot."

Joel walked us to the door. "I'll tell you," he said, "you wouldn't know Rochelle when she's straight. But when she's had some coke, she really changes. I've got to get her straightened out."

Lenny wrapped his arm around Joel's shoulder. "Listen, man," he said, "she loves you. You know that."

"I know," Joel said.

"If I can do anything to help," he said. "Anything at all. You just ask me. I don't care if it's three in the morning. Anything at all."

Joel hugged Lenny. "I know, man. Thanks. I really mean it."

In the car, the short distance back to the hotel, Lenny told me that he thought he was about to make a major deal with two men who were proprietors of sex-aids manufacturing companies who were very tight with the man who owned two adult book shops in the valley. "With a guy like Joel," he said, "you can make the kinds of contacts that count."

"I can see that," I said.

"This town is full of really beautiful people," Lenny said. "The kind of people who would do anything for you."

I thought of the faces of the people at Joel's party, the faces of the born graspers and manipulators of the world, and I thought of Lenny and Linda, two innocents in the lions' den, pretending to be lions. Then, when I got back to the Beverly Hills Hotel, I went into the Polo Lounge for a nightcap. The people in the dim bar looked so tough, so hardened, that I worried about what people who were not hard down to their toes could do to survive in Los Angeles.

But then, Lenny had just made $37,500 in one month. He was obviously at home here. I walked out by the pool and saw a beautiful woman swimming under the palm trees, with moonlight reflecting on the water. Perhaps this place is paradise after all, I thought. The woman climbed out of the pool, shook the water out of her hair, and walked past me into a cabana. She had long auburn hair and a wide, friendly smile. Yes, I thought, maybe this is the place.

Perhaps I had been wrong about Lenny all along. Perhaps he had not been confused about what he wanted. Perhaps he had really just wanted money and to be around people who were rich and had beautiful girl friends who were high all the time. Perhaps there was no conflict within him at all. He just wanted money and the good life, and now he would be happy. At least that was possible. He did seem extremely happy, after all.

As it happened, the story was far more complex than that. Lenny was stretching the rubber band inside him tighter and tighter, putting all of his bets on the number that said he could get all he ever wanted from life by making money in real-property tax shelters. He denied that any other part of him even existed. That was fine as long as the number kept paying off. But if it ever stopped, and the rubber band snapped back, where would Lenny be?

But, for the time being, the number kept paying off.

LOS ANGELES, 1976-1977
THE WILD WORLD

Snapshots of Lenny and Linda as the hot young couple in Los Angeles in the days when everything seemed possible:

In the summer of 1976, I moved out to Los Angeles on a fool's errand for a famous producer. My work at the studio took almost no time. I was mostly asked questions such as whether it would be possible to smuggle a rhinoceros into the boardroom of the Federal Reserve Board. The rest of my time was my own. One day in the late summer I went out with Lenny on a selling mission.

Cut into the hills on the side of the Hollywood Freeway was the beginning of a small shopping center. It is impossible for someone who has not lived in Los Angeles to imagine what a desolate scene it was. The sun was pouring down through a thick layer of smog. Not forty feet from where we stood, ten lanes of traffic sped by. The air was so foul from exhaust that nothing grew except a weedlike grass. Even that had been scooped away so that the ground lay exposed as raw and lifeless. The noise from the freeway was overwhelming, like the noise on an airport runway, but constant, never weakening. On the ground were beer bottles, Big Mac wrappers, an acre of broken glass, whole sections of the *Los Angeles Times*, baby bottles, old records, television sets, even sprung sofas. It was as if the freeway travelers had discarded every relic of daily life as they hurtled toward a new kind of life of permanent motion.

On this site was a small billboard which read, "Future Site of Paradise Cove Shopping Center."

Lenny pulled his Mercedes onto the ground. He pointed at various clumps of dead grass, particularly deep indentations in the ground, raised mounds of red dirt. "That's where the bank will be," he said. "That's where the drugstore will be. That's where the fish-'n'-chips place will be."

I looked at it all and wondered why anyone would want to work in a store right next to a freeway manufacturing poisonous gases.

Lenny shrugged his shoulders.

"The way we have this deal figured out," he said, "we're going to be making money from the moment we start. We're going to get a loan that's big enough to pay for all of the construction, all of the landscaping" (I gasped) "and then some boot which we just get to take home with us."

The investors showed up. They were airline pilots from United. They looked as if they had been stamped out of a plant for making wholesome-looking Americans. One was called "Buck," and the other was Bob. They looked beefy, contented, sure that the world was their oyster. Each man looked florid, as if he had been fishing in the Chattahoochee for two weeks before he showed up. Both men wore Hawaiian shirts and jeans. They asked a few questions in deep, serious tones. Then Buck said, "And what's the write-off in the second year?"

Lenny gave a long, involved answer, which the pilots listened to intently. He explained about tax courts and accountants' opinions, and then he looked at both men seriously and said, "I can only tell you that if this investment was not one hundred percent safe, I doubt very much that Mr. Van Swearingen would have invested in it."

The two pilots looked at each other and looked impressed. They signed the papers right there on the freeway shoulder, with one thousand cars going by every minute. After they left, Lenny told me that Van Swearingen was the board chairman of United Airlines.

"And he bought into this?" I asked.

"He absolutely did," Lenny said. "We gave him a full share for a half-share price so that we could tell all the pilots that he was in. Good idea, huh?"

The pilots invested sixty thousand each, and for that hour's work, Lenny made about four thousand dollars. If psychiatrists could have seen how happy Lenny was after making that much money, a whole new branch of medicine about the relation of people to money would have started, dwarfing Kohutian analysis in its scope.

"I'm telling you, man," he said, "this is the way I always knew it would be. You know what it feels like to pitch a deal to people and have them buy it? Do you know what it's like to have people take your word for something and then give you money because they trust you, they respect you? You know what that's like? It's great. That's what it's like."

Lenny looked as if he had been told that he would never again feel pain.

Snapshot two is in the baccarat room of Caesar's Palace. Lenny's friend Joel had taken ten of his closest friends in his brand-new Gulfstream II to fly for a night of revelry in Vegas. Joel had been feeling restless because the smog was bad. He called Lenny and asked him to come to Vegas for the evening. Lenny asked if he could bring me. "Of course," Joel said. "Do you think I fly around in a little Lear Jet or something?"

Linda came along. So did Rochelle and Michael and some other people in the auto-detailing business and the auto-parts business and the pinball-arcade business. All of the men looked like rabbinical students who had decided to make money instead. The girls all looked as if they would just as soon kill the men they were with as fuck them and vice versa.

Joel had arranged for three limousines to take us from McCarran Airport to Caesar's. I sat with Rochelle, Joel, Lenny, and Linda. Joel wore a pair of jeans and a starched white shirt. His thick, sulking lips were half open in a kind of anticipatory grin. He and Rochelle passed a gram bottle of cocaine back and forth, draining the container before we reached the hotel. Joel took another gram of cocaine out of his shirt pocket and hit up several more times before we got out of the car. He offered the drug to Lenny three times. Each time, Lenny turned it down.

By the time the limo pulled up in front of Caesar's, Joel was wired like an electric blackbird. His hands were shaking so badly he could not reach the door handle. The chauffeur opened the door. Joel bounded from the car and literally ran into the casino. Lenny ran along behind him. "He's my pal," Lenny said. "I have to be sure he's all right."

We followed through the dazzling casino to the baccarat table, which was separated from the main part of the room by a row of columns and a velvet rope. By the time we arrived, Joel was shaking hands with a pit boss in a tuxedo who looked as if his eyes could cut glass. The man was bald and well prepared for Joel.

"The usual limit is four thousand dollars per card," the pit boss said. "But for you, Mr. Miller, no limit, of course."

Joel nodded and sat down to play. Lenny looked utterly transfixed. He stared from Joel to the pit boss and back. This was really the big time. Those words, "For you, Lenny, no limit," were the words Lenny wanted to hear someday.

Rochelle looked at Joel and then took Lenny's arm. "What a fucking show-off," she said. "He won't even pay for his maid's social security," she added.

Lenny did not listen to her. He watched Joel throw thousand-dollar chips onto the table as if they were peanut shells. His face had a quality of longing that I had never seen before on an adult's face. Linda noticed it and grasped Lenny's other arm. "Let's look around," she said. "I've never been to Las Vegas. Maybe we'll see somebody famous."

Lenny did not budge. He just watched Joel gamble.

After a few minutes, Linda, Rochelle, and I walked around the casino. Caesar's is much quieter than most casinos. It aims for the high roller, rather than the slot-machine player. That means less noise. Rochelle drifted off to a twenty-dollar blackjack table. Linda and I went into the lounge and watched a comedian imitate an Italian priest.

"Lenny is losing weight," Linda said. "He's hustling around all the time. He hardly ever eats."

"That's because he's doing so well," I said.

"I wish he would eat more," she said. "I just think of him running all over town working so hard, and he never has enough to eat. He's always hungry." She shook her head and looked at the floor.

Lenny did not gamble on the trip. He just watched Joel and then looked sad on the airplane ride back.

Snapshot three. It was a Saturday afternoon. Lenny called me up. "I have a great surprise for Linda," he said. "I need your help."

Lenny and I drove over to a Jaguar dealer in West Los Angeles. There, in the middle of the lot, was a gleaming, sleek white Jaguar XJ6. It looked as if it was moving even when it was standing still. Lenny had some conversation with the dealer, a heavy Jewish man with an English accent. Then he signed a few forms. He also handed the man a certified check.

"You drive my car," he said. "You know how to drive a Mercedes. I'll drive Linda's car home."

When we got back to the house in the Hollywood Hills, Lenny hid Linda's car in the garage. He left his out on the street. He and I sat in the study watching a baseball game, a horse race, and a gymnastics contest on all three of Lenny's TV's. "See," he said, "I tried to think what I could get Linda for her birthday that would let her know that we've really arrived, that we really are at the place we've always wanted to be. So I thought of this car 'cause like I told you, once I saw this car in a James Bond movie, and I could see that Linda really liked it. So it's like part of a dream for her, really, which is how I would like for her to think of our entire life together. It's just like a dream. From now on it's all downhill."

Linda came home from ballet class in her rented car. I think it was a Valiant or a Pacer. She carried groceries out of the trunk into the kitchen. Her hair was longer and more beautiful than ever. Her dark blue eyes flashed with youth and energy. She smiled as if she meant it.

Lenny came out of the study and hugged her. He reached into a cabinet and took out a box of twelve red roses. "Happy birthday," he said. Then he kissed her. Out of an impromptu spirit of good fun, he started to sing, "Happy birthday to you." I joined in. As we sang, he waltzed Linda through the entrance hall, toward the bedroom, through the bedroom. into another hall, and then into the garage. With one hand around her shoulder and another on the light switch, he twirled Linda around, turned on the light, and showed her the Jaguar.

She shrieked, jumped up and down, and hugged Lenny as if she would squeeze him into herself. She pounded on the car's vinyl top, opened the door, felt the red leather seats, turned on the radio, beeped the horn, and even climbed into the back seat. She started to cry as she climbed out of the back seat into the garage. Lenny held her in his arms and hugged her. She cried great big tears of joy onto his shoulder. He held her in his arms and patted her on the back, as a father comforts a baby.

"I told you," he said to her. "I told you someday this would happen. I told you."

Snapshot four. This is a really small one. I was having dinner with Lenny and Linda at the Palm. Lenny said he would like to order another bottle of Piper-Heidsieck. "I don't know if you should, Lenny," Linda said. "Our American Express is a month overdue already."

Lenny smiled and said, "I'll put it on Master Charge."

"That's two months overdue," Linda said. "I don't need any more champagne. Do you, Ben?"

"I want more champagne," Lenny said. "I just haven't gotten to the bills. It's just because I've been so busy making money that I haven't had time to pay any of my bills."

We all ate our lobsters in silence for a minute, and then Lenny shook his head in disgust. "What's the point of really going out and doing something right if your wife still thinks you're a bum?"

Linda looked as if someone had struck her. "Lenny," she said. "Lenny."

Lenny looked angry for a moment, then smiled and chucked her under the chin. "You're right," he said. "I'll have some more champagne, and then I'll go right home and pay those bills."

Linda smiled and went back to her lobster, but when the waiter came, Lenny just ordered coffee and no champagne. He looked as if he had been chastened, which was a way Lenny did not like to look.

"I'm sorry, Lenny," Linda said. She took his hand. "I'm sorry. That was really stupid of me."

"It's OK," Lenny said. "It's OK."

I left in my own car and let them get on to their house alone together.

A man at the *Wall Street Journal* had once told me that even Saudi Arabia could spend money faster than it came in, but of course that is not the point of the story.

Snapshot number five. In the spring of 1977, Lenny and Linda rented a small beach house on Malibu Beach Road, just up the road from the Malibu Beach Colony. They had it for a few weeks, then Lenny made a particularly big haul on an apartment complex in Downey, and he was off to the races. He decided that they should have a house in the Colony itself. Right there with Lou Adler and all the moguls. He found a small house which fronted on the sand. It was next to a famous singer-songwriter's house. It had a small back-yard with a picket fence looking out on the blue Pacific.

One afternoon I sat in a web chair watching Lenny and Linda play in the ocean. It was a weekday. The beach was deserted. Two children dug a deep hole in the sand. An old man sat in a chair and tended a fishing pole. The ocean broke and refracted itself into a million different pieces, shining and then darkening in the afternoon sun. The waves came up in enormous rolls and then broke across the shoreline for as far as I could see. The waves crashed and resounded up and down the beach, a symphony of power and eternity.

Lenny wore a modest yellow bathing suit. Linda wore a stunning red one-piece. Her black hair glistened and shone in the sun. She climbed on his back while he carried her out to the waves. When a wave broke over them, she cried out and screamed with laughter. She fell into the surf, then climbed back up on Lenny's back and waited for the next wave. Sometimes she would slide around in front of Lenny and kiss him as the waves crashed on their heads. The wave would dissolve in white foam, and there would be Lenny and Linda, wobbling in the undertow, but still kissing.

I watched them for a half hour, listening to reports on the news about a golf tournament and about Bert Lance. Then they walked in from the surf, across the wide, sandy beach, hand in hand.

"That's pretty good," I said. "It looked like you were having a good time."

*

Linda hugged Lenny around the waist. "This is as good as it gets," she said.

The final snapshot. Christmas 1977 at Lenny and Linda's house on Hollywood Boulevard. Joel and Michael and Rochelle all went out of town to Puerto Vallarta for the holiday. It brought them down to be in town at such a sentimental time. So Joel had his G-II take everyone to Puerto Vallarta, where he had a row of cottages at a famous hotel.

Joel told Lenny that if he and Linda changed their minds and decided to join the party, Lenny only needed to call. "I'll tell that lazy bastard who flies my plane, and he'll be up for you in a hot second."

Lenny offered to send Linda home for the holidays to her parents' farm in western Massachusetts. "I can't get away," he told her. "There's a lot of foreigners who come into town over the holidays, and they all want into American land deals because they all have American income to shelter. I could make a lot of money before New Year's."

Linda would not go without Lenny. "This is our first Christmas that we've ever spent when we've been really sure we're on the right track, when we knew where we were going. Let's spend it together."

"What about last year?" Lenny asked.

"Last year you were sure, but I wasn't completely sure," she said. This conversation took place at Ma Maison, where I had come along with my new wife. Jerry Brown, like some weird doppelgänger, was at the next table with Gray Davis.

So on Christmas Day, Lenny and Linda were alone in their house, opening presents under a tree while the sun shone dazzlingly outside the windows and the pool lay invitingly under a jacaranda tree. My wife and I came to give them our presents. I gave Lenny a starter's pistol. My wife gave Linda a machete because she was always complaining about the rapid growth of the palms next to the kitchen. I cannot remember what they gave us. We all ate a ham dinner that Linda had made. Then we sat and talked about L.A. life.

"You know, I had a man come to me to buy into a syndicate, and the guy brought seventy-five thousand dollars in cash?" Lenny said.

"So I asked him what kind of business he was in. The guy looks at me without batting an eye and tells me he's in the narcotics division of the L.A.P.D."

Linda talked about the men in her ballet class. "They're mostly gay black men," she said, "but they're perfectly nice to me. I just don't like it that much when they start giggling. It's real distracting." She wore jeans and a cotton shirt. She ran her fingers through her black hair and then shook her head. The sunlight streamed through her hair.

"You won't have to worry about it for long," Lenny said. "I'm going to rent you your own ballet studio. I would've done it already if I had time."

Linda looked down at the mass of wrapping paper, shirts, bracelets, stereo tapes, necklaces, and a camera on the floor under the tree. "You've given me so much," she said. "Too much." She took Lenny's hand. "And the presents are the least of it."

Lenny shook his head. "I told you I would get you your own ballet studio, and I will," he said.

She took his hand in both of hers and squeezed it. "One squeeze," she said. She squeezed it again. "Two squeezes," she said. She squeezed it a third time. "Three squeezes," she said. "I love you."

Lenny smiled at her, then said, "Oh, I have to get some papers out of my car. Just a second."

He ran out of the room to the garage. In a moment, he was back with a huge box, wrapped in red paper, with a few air holes in the side. "I almost forgot this," he said.

Tears came to Linda's eyes. "Lenny, you didn't," she said. She tore the wrapping and the box. Inside was a black cocker spaniel puppy. The puppy cried and jumped into Linda's arms. She hugged it and started to shake. She was so happy she was literally shaking with joy.

The puppy peed on her blouse, but she didn't care. Lenny stood over her as she knelt with the puppy, making a tableau of a happy young family.

That is the last snapshot in the album of Lenny and Linda as the couple on the move.

LOS ANGELES, SPRING 1978
THE CHUTE

You might think that people make their own problems. Perhaps they do, but it takes two to have an accident. In Lenny's case, he was one of the two. The other one was a bureaucrat in the Treasury Department in Washington, D.C., whom Lenny has never met. That faceless man or woman began the whole thing, although Lenny surely was carrying around his own vial of hemlock all through his life. If you take a guy like Lenny who is completely dependent on how much money he makes, who his friends are, what kind of car he has, how he is doing in the minute-by-minute competition with his peers, you have a man with one foot already in the grave.

There was Lenny, for two years riding along on the big wave of accomplishment in the real-estate tax-sheltered syndication business. Inside him was a shark of self-loathing and self-hate. If that shark did not get fed a daily dose of achievement and money, it would become hungry for Lenny's soul, for his life itself. If the beast could not be appeased by steady feedings of getting the right table at La Scala and having his car parked right out front by the valets at Mr. Chow, that beast would have Lenny's heart instead. The shark was never appeased, never had enough. Lenny could feed it half a million dollars' worth of syndication sales in one day. The shark would be just as ravenous the next day. Lenny could shove a white Jaguar for his wife into the shark's maw, and the shark would only want to know what Lenny had done for it lately.

70

Some might say that Lenny should have killed that shark a long time ago. He should have stopped feeding the monster and shown himself that he could survive even with the shark gnawing at his guts, until the shark died of neglect. But Lenny did not become the kind of man who can live without constantly assuaging the anger within him. Like almost everyone in Los Angeles, he became the slave to his own demands for proof that he deserved to live. Without that daily proof, he was a dead man.

For two years, the proof came in buckets. Lenny could do no wrong. The shark was fed, slept for a day, and Lenny could rest and feel joy. He told the truth when he told me and everyone else how happy he was. For the first time in his life, he had drugged the creature of self-loathing. He could go about his business without pausing every moment to hate himself for his failures. A man who feels no blows of low self-esteem is a happy man. That was Lenny for almost two years.

And then there was Linda. She had never expected to accomplish much. In a blessed way, she accepted herself as a human being who deserved to have some small space on the planet. If she simply went about her business going to ballet, shopping with her friends, meeting people to raise money for lost cats and dogs, she was content. If she had a roof over her head and clothing to wear and three squares a day, that was enough. She had no demon whipping her to feed it with money and position.

Of course, she was extremely concerned with every detail of Lenny's life. If he was not happy, she was not happy. If he felt like a bum, she felt sad that he felt that way. But her feelings were the feelings of a loving woman toward a man who is in pain. She felt sympathetic, but she could not possibly approximate the extent of Lenny's anguish when the creature of self-contempt was tearing away at Lenny's soul.

On the other hand, she could not feel the limit of his ecstasy at finally having satisfied the beast for a long time. He was soaring with euphoria. She was more quietly content with what she saw as her Lenny's long overdue ascent to his proper place in the world.

Then came that man at the Treaury Department, who had never heard Lenny's name and had no idea of what was about to happen to a man who had known happiness for the first time in his life, all because the bureaucrat had a thought about how to tighten up a portion of the Internal Revenue Code relating to the allowance of an investment tax credit for limited partners in real-property transactions. Probably one day the GS-13 sat at the Treasury Department cafeteria enjoying a Mighty Mo triple-decker cheeseburger when he told the man next to him that he had an idea. In that dimly lit enormous room, the two men talked about how the investment tax credit is meant to reward investors who gamble and build new buildings. It certainly was not meant to allow doctors and dentists and airline pilots to avoid their fair tax burden.

The two men probably wrote a memo about it after lunch, had their secretary type it, then sent it to the head of their division. As I see it, the head of the division was at a conference on taxation in the Virgin Islands. But his assistant, a hot young law grad from Georgetown with a master's in taxation, got the memo. The assistant thought that he had a piece of dynamite in his hands which would surely go right to the head of the column about tax developments in every Tuesday's *Wall Street Journal* (you see what a small world this is). As it happened, the assistant's girl friend lived in a house in the old section of Alexandria, Virginia, where the cute old houses have been restored so that it looks almost like Georgetown. One of the roommates in the house was a girl who was just starting out in the Washington office of the *Wall Street Journal* after studying journalism at the University of Maryland. So the assistant in the IRS figured that he could definitely make some brownie points with his girl friend if he gave the hot scoop to the roommate that the IRS was considering blowing real-estate tax shelters right out of the water. He picked up his telephone to make a call. It took so long for him to get an outside line that he figured he would forget the whole damned thing and tell his girlfriend about it the next night when they were supposed to go to Wolf Trap to see a local ballet troupe from Baltimore perform *Swan Lake* under the stars. Maybe that would persuade her to spend the night at his new apartment.

Meanwhile, Lenny is still roaring along the highway of success at a dazzling pace, just as if he were careening along a freeway bridge utterly unaware that the bridge stopped in midair about two miles farther on. It was April in Los Angeles. That year was the worst year for rains in thirty years. Torrents of warm Pacific water poured down on Los Angeles for weeks on end. The sides of hills in Hollywood and Brentwood slid down onto half-million-dollar homes.

Water backed up in the Los Angeles River, normally a dry concrete culvert. A little boy from Studio City drowned trying to recover his bicycle in the river. Traffic on the San Bernardino Freeway was stop-and-go for ten days as huge lakes spread across all twelve lanes near West Covina.

That did not even slow down Lenny and Max Sherman. They paid some putz at the UCLA Art Department to make scale models of their projects. There were neat little shopping centers under plexiglass, adorable little apartment complexes with plastic grass (and no freeway garbage) right on tables in Century City, meticulously accurate artists' renderings of office buildings perfect down to the license plates of the Porsche painted in front of the building (PROFITS, read the plate). The investors strolled into the offices of Century West Equities, sat down, had a drink with Lenny and Max, and heard about how they were going to save taxes and get rich while they lounged in leather chairs forty floors above the pavement.

In 1978, real-estate prices were rising so fast that a buyer could see the price of a house going up right in front of his eyes, like a miracle grass that grew to a man's height in a day. Buyers appeared out of every corner of the world to plunk down their money in any corner of southern California where there was still room to build or buy. Lenny could not get the lawyers to write up his prospectuses fast enough to accommodate all the investors. Century West Equities had the printers working night shifts to get out their brochures. But people would have bought without any prospectuses or brochures. The market had now reached the stage where word of mouth spread from Beverly Hills to Caracas to Tehran to Mexico City to Deauville to Rye to Buenos Aires to wherever people had money and wanted to see it grow and not pay taxes on it. Old women in babushkas speaking only Farsi wandered into Century West Equities and plunked down their money. Heads of newly appointed African states in long robes pulled up in limousines and handed over Mark Cross attaché cases filled with stacks of hundred-dollar bills. Little old Jewish couples, each one of whom had a small chain of hardware stores in Ohio, came in, cursed the rain for making their feet hurt, and signed checks for $250,000.

"There's no law against getting rich," Lenny told me one night at dinner at La Scala. "Everybody who isn't crazy wants to get rich."

I was in a constant transport of envy, so I agreed with every word

Lenny had to say. By now even I, a thoroughly frightened person where money is concerned, hoped one day to have Lenny take my pitiful savings and make me rich.

Linda picked at her canelloni and said that she was sure that when the rain stopped Lenny would do even better. "After all," she said, "who wants to look at real estate when it's raining?"

Lenny laughed with his mouth full of cream of vegetable soup. "It doesn't matter if there's an earthquake," he said. "There's nothing that can stop people when they're convinced that they're going to make money. We could have a volcanic eruption, and people would still be dying to get their money down to make a few bucks. People are so crazy to get in on L.A. real estate that they'd walk through a world war to get in on it."

Lenny made a funny face at the foursome in the booth across the room. At the table were two men who looked like yeshiva *buchers* in Pierre Cardin suits without ties and two women wearing leather trousers so tight you could have used them to stop arterial bleeding.

"The guy on the right is really big in plastic love dolls," Lenny said. "He is like the king of life-size sex aids. It's really an incredible story."

"How long can this go on with the real estate?" I asked Lenny. "How long can it keep going up like crazy? Is there anything else in history that has always gone up and never come down?"

Lenny looked at me as if I were crazy. "Are you kidding, Benjy?" he asked. "How high is up? What reason is there for this real-estate boom to ever end? Especially if you can skip out on your taxes at the same time? What's to make it ever go down? Everyone wants to live in L.A. Everyone wants to pay no taxes. What's ever gonna make it go down?"

Lenny excused himself for a moment to go over to talk to the largest factor in life-size sex aids, the John D. Rockefeller of dildoes. Linda touched my arm. "Lenny's put down a deposit on his own plane. It's just a propeller one, a Citation, but he's really excited about it."

"Does he know how to fly?" I asked.

"No, but he'll get someone to fly it for him," Linda said. "He's too busy making money to learn how to fly."

She was beginning to sound like him. I remembered a boy in my high school class named Sonny Jackson. He was a fine ball player.

When he graduated, he got $25,000 to sign with the Colt .45's, an expansion team in Houston. He went out and bought a Chevrolet Impala and had it driven around the parking lot at the local drive-in restaurant by a friend because he did not have a driver's license. I have not heard of Sonny Jackson in fifteen years.

Two nights after we went to La Scala, Lenny had his pilot fly Linda and Joel and Rochelle and me to Cabo San Lucas in his Citation. It was a bumpy flight because a prop plane cannot fly as high as a jet. The seats were covered with torn vinyl, compared with Joel's sheepskin seat covers on his G-II. There was no wet bar or refrigerator.

"I'm just sort of trying it out," Lenny told Joel, "just to see if I'd really like having my own plane."

Joel smiled at him paternally and said, "It's fine, Lenny, just fine."

In Cabo San Lucas, Joel and Lenny went to look at a discotheque at a new hotel. They were considering buying in. "It takes a hundred thousand to get in the bidding," Joel said to Lenny. "That's a lot of money."

Lenny clapped Joel on the back and winked. "I think I can swing it," he said.

"It's nonrefundable if you back out," Joel said.

"I don't back out of things, Joel," Lenny said.

"I know that's the kind of guy you are," Joel said.

"I feel as if like it's time to diversify," Lenny said. "I think I'd like to go into leisure-time activities. That's obviously where the next boom is coming."

"I think so," Joel said. "After all, people are going to have more and more money and are going to be working less and less. So they'll have to have something to do. And somebody's going to make some money out of it and that might as well be us, instead of some goys at some big company in New York."

"I'll give you the check for a hundred thousand as soon as we get back to L.A.," Lenny said. His eyes looked noticeably warm. Linda looked at Lenny as if she might speak, but she said nothing.

We went into the Imperador Hotel for dinner. Lenny had the limousine wait for us so that we could get back to the airport right after dinner. The entire point of flying to a place like Cabo San Lucas for dinner is that you get back the same night, so that it does not seem as if you were going on a weekend excursion like a retired postal clerk from San Diego. Lenny had learned a thing or two from

Joel. Through a Spanish-speaking woman at Century West Equities, Lenny had arranged for the captain to give us a special curtained-off room in the restaurant, far from where the Three-Star Tour Groups ate their choice of steak or lobster. Our room looked out over the ocean. Huge waves broke over the sand, then dissolved into an infinity of surging white bubbles, then floated slowly up onto the beach. Powerful halogen lights outside the hotel lit up the foam. The waves were so loud that they drowned out the mariachi music coming from the tourist room. I wished that Lenny were selling tax-sheltered participations in the waves. They would really last forever.

Between courses, Lenny watched Joel fill his nostrils with cocaine, then pass the bottle to Rochelle. She dipped a small spoon into the bottle at first and then inhaled the drug into her nostrils. After an hour, she simply used her long fingernails. Lenny and Linda did not take any of the drug. Instead, they lifted toast after toast of Piper champagne (their new favorite) to congratulate themselves and everyone they knew for the fabulous good fortune they had enjoyed to get into Los Angeles and meet such fine people as Joel and Rochelle ("You'll meet a lot of faggots here," Rochelle said); to get into southern California real estate at just the moment that the whole world realized that it was the best buy in history; to meet up with Max Sherman; and to be alive, young, and rich.

Joel was far too wired to respond with anything but a tightly stretched grin and a nod of his head. Rochelle smiled at Lenny the way a mother smiles at a little boy playing with his pet dog. She knows that the dog is likely to die before the little boy and that the little boy will suffer for it. Every so often she shook her head as if to ask herself how anyone could be such a fool.

Naturally, Joel kept going to the bathroom. After the third time he left, Rochelle stretched like a particularly clever cat and smiled at Lenny. "If you give him a dime for that disco you're out of your mind," she said. "You think you're going into it on the same terms he is? Are you crazy?"

"Please, Rochelle," Lenny said. "I trust Joel. He's played very square with me. The coke is making you talk like that."

"The fuck it is," Rochelle said. "Look, Lenny, there's something about you I like. I can't stand it that you're going to get fucked over like this by a creep like Joel."

"I'm sure Lenny knows how to protect himself," Linda said.

Rochelle turned and looked at Linda. She raised her eyebrows and shook her head. "If you think so," Rochelle said, "you're in for a hell of a surprise, yutzel."

"Let's not talk about this anymore," Lenny said. "I don't even like to talk behind Joel's back at all."

Rochelle looked at him intently. Her eyes looked sad. Then she shrugged her shoulders and sniffed more cocaine.

In the limousine, on the way back to the Citation, Lenny and Joel talked about liquor licenses, average cost per drink, maintenance costs, bribes to the *federales*, utilities, and all the other minutiae of owning a discotheque in Cabo San Lucas.

"Of course, the big bucks will come in the winter," Joel said. "We have to decide right off the bat whether we want to give a special rate for tour groups."

Lenny nodded appraisingly. "I expect this operation to be in the black from day one," he said. "I would bet that we would get all of our money out of it in the first year," he added.

Joel said, "Well, I think so, but we can't be sure."

Lenny said, "Joel, I think people like you and me don't go into deals that we don't know are sure things. Do you? I don't think either of us is looking for a passbook savings account. Right?"

"It could be very big," Joel said. "Cabo San Lucas is going to be far bigger than Puerto Vallarta."

"I think so," Lenny said. "In fact, I don't see why we need to get any other partners into this thing, to tell the truth. Why don't you and I just go into it ourselves? Why should we give any of it away?"

"Well, Mike's already put in a hundred fifty thousand. You could buy him out," Joel said, "but he'd want some profit for putting in his money. I'd think that with him and a few others, you'd be in for about half a million."

Even in the darkened interior of the plane, Lenny looked pale. In a slightly lower voice, he said, "I think we might be able to swing it." Linda gasped and turned away. I could see she clutched her purse.

Joel said, "It might be a little rich for you. I don't want you to go into it if it means that you and Linda are going to be eating baked beans from now on."

Lenny squared his shoulders, laughed, and said, "I think I can swing it. I'll give you the first hundred thousand when we get back. I'll have to sell some CD's to get the rest."

Joel slapped his hand on the arm of the seat. "I told you, everybody. This guy is so hot he's smoking. He's going to make the rest of us look like welfare mothers."

In the darkness of the cabin, I could see Lenny take deep breaths as if to fill himself up for his new role as man of property. I thought of Soames Forsyte, risking his life before the gods by daring to leave his nest and become a man of property. Now here was Lenny, twenty-four months ago a subway rider, today traveling in his own airplane. Twenty-four months ago he was unemployed and nearly broke. Now he was plunking down money in hundred-thousand-dollar lumps to buy into a discotheque in Cabo San Lucas in a hotel that was not even open yet. But Soames Forsyte had a wealthy father and grandfather, a prosperous law practice, enough money to live on the interest for the rest of his life. Lenny had a smile and a shoeshine and the absolute moral certainty that people would want to buy tax-sheltered investments from him for the rest of his life.

Soames Forsyte became a man of property when he could easily afford it. Lenny Brown was about to become a man of property on the come. Soames Forsyte bought a plot of land in suburban London, then the most important metropolis in the world. Lenny Brown bought a murky interest in a yet-to-be-open discotheque on the southern tip of Baja California.

If I told this to Lenny, he would have said that Soames Forsyte had not learned how much money could be made in the sheltering of personal income from federal tax.

A week later, Lenny asked me to come with him and Linda to an address on Melrose Boulevard where they were thinking of making yet another investment. A small building housing a stationery store and an upholstery shop was for sale. It was not particularly interesting, except that above the stores it had a small dance studio. At present, the studio was used to warehouse bolts of cloth for seat covers. But the hardwood floor was still there. So were the barres and the mirrors. There was a row of windows along one side, coated with dust, but they, like everything, could be cleaned.

Linda was giggling with excitement and anticipation. She was eager to have her own studio, but reluctant to lure Lenny further down the path of financial encumbrance. She wore her hair in a chignon, though, and a leotard top, as if she could not stop herself from dressing like a ballet mistress. Her dark blue eyes shone in the dusty studio.

"It's an awful lot of money," Linda said. "It would be wonderful, but it's an awful lot of money. I'm getting along perfectly fine at the Danceworks. It's really an extravagance." Still, she wrung her hands with excitement.

"The landlord's a Hungarian bandit," Lenny said. "He says I have to buy the whole building, and he wants half cash down. It comes to about a hundred seventy-five thousand in cash."

Linda clapped her hands to her face. "Oh, Jesus, that's too much money," she said. "I had no idea it was that much. Let's just forget about it." She pulled him by the elbow, as if to leave the building, to tear him and her away from temptation and disaster. Her small features were set, determined, and still there was a tentative edge to her voice.

Lenny smiled and laughed his laugh which was supposed to show that he was confident beyond what anyone else might dream of. "Just a minute," he said, shaking loose Linda's hand. "It's not just for amusement. This whole area is going to get upgraded. This is going to be very valuable land. There's not much doubt of that. I expect to make money in this place while you're dancing."

"I don't want us to get in over our heads," Linda said. "It doesn't do us any good at all if this place goes up if we're broke."

Lenny scowled and stamped his foot like a child. "Even after all this, you still think I'm a bum," he said. "I'm making money so fast they can't keep track of it over at Max's, and everybody in this town thinks I'm doing really well and my wife thinks I'm a bum."

He turned and faced the wall in a pout. Linda walked over to him and hugged him, pressing her face into his back. "It's not that at all," she said. "You're incredibly successful. I think you're the most successful man I've ever heard of. I just don't want you to feel like you're on a treadmill, having to make more and more money just to pay for things we've bought that we don't really need."

Lenny wheeled around and said, "Linda, I guarantee you the whole thing is incidental. The way things are going, we won't miss the money this costs, and meanwhile, I promised it to you a long time ago. So you should have it."

"I just know that sometimes you get bored with things and you don't want to do them anymore, and I don't want us to get into that situation and find that we owe everybody a lot of money when you don't want to work anymore," Linda said.

"Hey, Linda," Lenny said, "wake up. That was when I had all those dead-end jobs where nobody thought big. Now that I'm in a place where I can get something done, where people think big, where I'm making a lot of money, I'm never going to get bored. This is just the beginning. There's no reason I shouldn't be a partner of Joel's and a partner in Century West and have my own construction business, too. Why shouldn't I? I'm pretty good at this."

Lenny and Linda went over to the Hungarian bandit's house near Fairfax. The man wore a skullcap and dressed in Hasidic clothes. He took a ten-thousand-dollar deposit from Lenny and said he wanted the rest of the money in ten days. He had a furrowed brow and pockmarks from acne all over his face. He looked like a Los Angeles Fagin. Lenny handed the man the check, and then we all went over to Little Tony's in North Hollywood for a pizza.

We slurped down the greasy food, and Lenny virtually glowed with pride. He was surrounded by men and women who had come in vans, who could not even imagine owning property, and he, Lenny Brown, had just bought an entire building in Los Angeles for his wife to use for a ballet studio or for any other damn thing she pleased. Linda was so excited that she couldn't eat. She talked about how she could now go to the studio and do ballet anytime she wanted. "If I felt like going at three in the morning, I could go, and there wouldn't be anyone to stop me." She spoke so loudly that a Mexican family at the next table stared at us. I had never known her to speak so loudly. Lenny kept getting up to put money into the juke box. He played every Rolling Stones song on the machine, because he loved them and they reminded him of when he was in college and everybody else was so snotty and he knew deep down inside that someday he was going to blow every one of them right out of the water. The music had just the quality of aggression he felt toward a doubting, vanquished world.

"If those faggots who used to come into Bloomingdale's and act like their asses were made of gold could see me now, could see that in a few years I could buy the whole store, they'd be pretty goddam amazed," he said.

"I'll bet," I said.

"Yes," he said as he ate a huge hunk of pizza, "they'd be pretty amazed because now I'm the one who could buy and sell them."

"If I feel like dancing on the Fourth of July, there's nobody to stop me," Linda said.

"You can't always get what you want," Mick Jagger said, "but if you try sometime, you just might find, you get what you need."

Meanwhile, as I imagine it, back in Washington, the assistant department chief in the Internal Revenue Service had just taken his girl friend to a really fancy meal at Nathan's. She was acting like she was going to go crazy if she didn't figure out some way to calm her roommate down, because the bitch was so jacked up trying to get stories that she was smoking all over the house, leaving ashtrays filled with dead cigarette butts all over the kitchen, borrowing other people's clothes that didn't belong to her and returning them smelling of cigarettes and perspiration, and frankly it made some people with neater habits a little sick.

So the assistant department chief suddenly remembered that he was sitting on a big story that the *Wall Street Journal* would just love to have. A new reporter like the roommate would freak out to get this inside dope. The young lawyer probably told his girl friend that the roommate should call him. The next day, the roommate does call, and the assistant department chief says that she first had to promise that she will not tell where she heard this amazing story. The roommate swears. Then the assistant department chief says that it so happens that the IRS is considering disallowing the investment tax credit for limited partners in real-estate-development partnerships.

"Huh?" says the roommate. They don't teach about ITC's in journalism school.

The assistant department chief explains what it means. She still doesn't get it. He blurts out, "It means it'll kill real-estate tax shelters."

That is the part that got into the *Wall Street Journal*'s tax-report column on a Tuesday in the spring or early summer of 1978. The item began, in bold-face type, "Demise of Real-Estate Tax Shelters?"

Then it continued that the IRS was "mulling" discontinuing the investment tax credit for limited partners in real-estate-development schemes. "The move would unquestionably have a negative effect on the popular real-estate tax-shelter deals that have become so widespread in recent years, especially in California."

Lenny did not get the *Wall Street Journal*. He only read it when it was passed around the fortieth-floor office of Century West Equities. When Lenny drove to work on that Tuesday, he was kicking himself for not having bought the building next to the dance studio building, too. The West Hollywood area was definitely in for major reconstruction, and after that would come Hollywood. The whole area around Melrose could become another Robertson Boulevard, with big office buildings and display houses. He vowed that the first thing he would do when he got to the office would be to call the county recorder's office and find out what the ownership story was on that old building next door.

In the elevator going up to the fortieth floor, Lenny also made a mental note to call Joel and ask him who the best dealer was for a Gulfstream II. Of course, Lenny couldn't afford even to come close to buying one yet, but it would be really good for Joel to think that Lenny was in that league. There was absolutely no reason, as far as Lenny could see, that a man who earned as much as he did and would in the future should have any qualms about getting his reputation around, even if he was a little short that month and had been getting really nasty calls from American Express.

If Joel thought that Lenny was in the G-II league, he would throw a helluva lot more business Lenny's way. That was the way of the world. Then the young moguls in boat insurance and time shares in Breckenridge condominiums would be paying up the money so that Lenny could have a G-II pretty soon.

Anyway, fuck American Express. They were in their big white building in lower Manhattan, each person in some damned little cubbyhole, each person leading his own really small life. They were in for six percent vig right off the top on each bill, so how the hell did they get the nerve to think that they should get paid right on the button the first minute someone gets a bill? When Lenny was really riding high, he would start his own American Express company, only it would cater to really successful young executives, and it would just discreetly charge them interest instead of nudging them as if they were coal miners in debt at the company store.

Lenny told me about two years later that he had had all those thoughts as he went up to the fortieth-floor offices of Century West Associates. The first thing he noticed when he went in the door was that it was unusually quiet. Most times, by ten in the morning, the telephones were ringing off the hook. This time, the receptionist sat at her desk reading the View section of the *Los Angeles Times*. She moved her thick lips as she read about a special "rap" group for abused Jewish housewives.

The sunlight poured into the office windows, bleaching out the textured wallpaper and the simulated antique magazine tables along the wall. Lenny went into his office. There was a note on his desk from Max Sherman. "Lenny. Please come in to see me ASAP."

Max looked unusually fat and sallow, seated behind his Louis XV desk, with his corner windows shaded by heavy burlap curtains. He had a bagel with cream cheese on a piece of white wax paper in front of him. He also had a copy of the *Wall Street Journal*. He was not wearing his usual cowboy tie, although he was wearing a cowboy shirt.

"So," Max said, "since when do you come in here at ten in the morning as if this were a bank?"

Lenny was taken aback by his tone. "I always come in around ten, Max," Lenny said. "That way, if people call me, it seems more like I'm a banker."

Lenny wondered what Max was so jacked up about.

"Max," Lenny said, "what's wrong? Did one of the deals fall through? We have a complaint from the government? What is it?"

Max, who was a movie fan, simply picked up the *Wall Street Journal* and tossed it to Lenny. It fell on the floor in front of him. He picked it up and saw the item Max had circled. It began, "Demise of Real-Estate Tax Shelters." Lenny did not understand why Max was so cranky. The article did not say anything about a new law. It just said that the IRS was "mulling" this idea. Anyway, the ITC wasn't the only good part of the deal.

"I don't get it," Lenny said. "It's just a rumor, and anyway, even if it happened, our lawyers could think of a new way around it. And not only that, people are buying in just for the profits now, not just for the tax shelter." Lenny could see that he was going to have to pull Max through this mess.

"You don't get it?" Max Sherman asked, rising from the table. His face reddened. "I'll tell you what there is to get. I've been on the phone for an hour talking to prospects, and no one is even returning my calls. So far this morning, while you were acting like some *meshuganah* banker, my secretary has taken eleven calls from investors who want out. Three lawyers for investors have called, saying that if they don't have their deposits back by this afternoon, they're cancelling the checks or suing or some goddam thing. I have three calls from lawyers at Manatt alone." Max Sherman sat back down in his chair. "Now are you starting to get it?" he asked.

"Max," Lenny said, "somebody has to explain to these people that this is just a rumor. Let's get on the phones right away and get this straightened out."

"We'd better," Max said. "We're on the hook for options on that property on La Cienega. If we don't get buyers for the deal, we eat that money. And that was a lot of money."

"I'm hip," Lenny said. He knew that he and Max and the other guys at Century West would not see any paychecks for a good long while if they didn't get investors to bail them out of the option on the La Cienega property. But Lenny also knew that he was a hot guy. He could sell refrigerators to Eskimos. He would make a few suave, sincerely meant telephone calls, and before you could say, "Ma Maison," the deal would be made and Max would stop bawling.

Lenny winked at Max. Max shook his head in disgust. Lenny said, "Max, in two hours you'll wonder what all the crying was about." Max threw up his hands and spun around his chair so that he could look out at the city, which went on about its business totally oblivious to the fate which had overtaken Lenny and Max and the other packagers of tax-sheltered equities.

Lenny adjusted himself in his Breuer chair, swallowed a few gulps of Perrier so that he would sound smooth and easy, and made his first call, to a very hot prospect who had said he would buy in for a hundred thousand to the development on La Cienega. The client was a young gynecologist in Santa Monica. The client said that he was really sorry but that his lawyer had warned him off the deal and had told him, in fact, that he would do well just to put the money in the bank and pay the tax, rather than get involved in something which might get him in real trouble down the road. "I'm just a doctor, Lenny," the hot prospect said. "I have to do what my lawyer tells me."

The second hot prospect was an Iranian exile who had taken about ten million dollars out of the country before he came to the good old U.S.A. When Lenny called to ask about dotting the i's and crossing the t's on his participation in the La Cienega project, the Iranian said, "Very sorry. My funds are tied up, Lenny. I cannot get at them right now. Very sorry."

Lenny would have argued with him, but just then, Lenny's secretary, Mary Pat, told him that there were three calls waiting. The first one was from the two airline pilots who had wanted in if Van Swearingen was in. Now they wanted to know if they could sell out. The second was from an orthodontist in Westwood who wanted to know if he could get out of a warehouse deal in Santa Ana. The third was from a reporter for *New West*. He wanted to do an Intelligencer gossip item about the death of the real-estate tax-shelter business. "Are you looking into the gold-coin business now?" he asked.

For the rest of the morning Lenny made one telephone call after another, took one telephone call after another. Proctologists from Reseda, appliance dealers from Cucamonga, roofing contractors from El Monte, every person who had been burning to give Lenny money now wanted his money back. Dress designers from the garment center, jewelry salesmen from downtown, even the policeman, wanted their money back. None of them came right to the point and said that he did not trust Lenny's deals anymore. There was always another reason. A sudden illness. An opportunity to get in on a stock when it came out. An unexpected tax payment. But the message was the same all morning long. The bubble had burst.

Professors from U.S.C. Petroleum engineers from Union Oil. Rug dealers from Iraq. Druggists from Hollywood. Business managers of TV stars. Trial lawyers. From all walks of life they told Lenny that they were not going through with the deals they had promised to go into.

By noon, Lenny was soaking wet. He had sweated through his shirt and his trousers even though the air-conditioning was set at sixty-five, in violation of federal law. His hands were trembling. He felt feverish and clammy at the same time. A dull pain spread across his chest. He had stitches of agony in his back. Mary Pat sent out for a corned beef sandwich on rye, which was Lenny's favorite. It lay uneaten on his desk all through the day.

At three o'clock, when he had struck out in almost fifty telephone calls, he walked into Max's office. Lenny was startled to see that Max looked far more relaxed than he had earlier in the day. Just that sight cheered Lenny up. He figured that the old fox had figured an angle that would carry the day. Maybe there had even been a story somewhere saying that business in the *Journal* was wrong.

"What's up, Lenny," Max asked. "Did you get any takers?"

"Not yet," Lenny said. "People are spooked. But you know, just the fact that everybody's so panicked and got panicked so fast tells me that people are going to get unpanicked just as fast." Lenny pulled himself together and threw back his shoulders. "I feel as if by tomorrow, the tide will definitely be turning our way again. In a week, people'll be beating down our doors again."

"Is that what you think, Lenny?" Max asked, raising his eyebrows and smiling.

"That's what I think," Lenny said.

Max suddenly slammed his palms down on his desk so hard that the noise made Lenny wince. "You poor kid," Max said through clenched teeth. "You poor, poor kid. What the hell gives you any idea about this kind of thing? I've been in this business for fifteen years. This is the coldest I've ever seen it. The stone-coldest."

"It's got to pick up," Lenny said.

"Why?" Max asked. "Why does it have to?"

"Because everyone wants California real estate," Lenny said.

"Yeah," Max said. "But they don't want it from us with us taking twenty percent off the top unless it's got the tax hook. If it doesn't have that, why should they buy an outhouse from us?"

That one really stumped Lenny. He started to sweat again. Max, who was not a mean person, leaned back in his chair and said, "Look, don't feel that bad. You're partly right about the whole thing."

Lenny snapped upward in his seat. He stared at Max, at the photos of Max's wife (Shelly) and his children (Mark and Steve) on the wall behind Max.

"We've had scares before, although not this bad. The fact is that it takes a few weeks, but things usually start to perk up again after a month, and we could easily be back to normal again in three months, six at the outside," Max said. "In the meantime, you've got a lot of money stashed away, I suspect, and you can just take it easy until things pick up again. Think of it as a sort of vacation."

"You mean we won't get any money coming in for maybe six months?" Lenny asked.

Max laughed. "Not only that, pal," he said, "but we're all going to have to go into the piggy bank for that option on the La Cienega property, and we're going to have to kick in for the overhead here, too."

"Why?" Lenny asked. "Why do we have to have this office going if we aren't going to be doing any selling?"

"Because, pal," Max said, "if we just fold up our tents and go off into the desert, people will think we're a two-bit operation, which we definitely are not. And if we don't keep the office open, how will anybody find us when the lawyers figure out some way around this thing or when the fucks in Washington decide they were just playing with their putzes? How will they ever find us to start investing in us again?"

Lenny looked ashen. Max got up and patted him on the back. "It ain't that bad, pal," he said. "You'll see. In a year, we'll be back up to full speed."

Then Max combed his hair and walked out of the room. "Think of it as a vacation," he said. "Just take some time off to think." He walked down the hall, but then he turned and came back. "By the way, pal," he said, "I've been letting the rent slide at your place because we were doing so well. But now I think it's probably time for you to start paying the rent. I think it's about two grand a month. Not too much of a strain for a guy who's been making it the way you have."

Lenny was shaking by now. Drops of perspiration were falling off his fingertips onto the Karastan rug in Max's office. He looked at his watch. It was only three-thirty. Plenty of time to make more calls. He could do it. He could, just by the sheer force of his need and his longing, break through and make those people buy into the deals. The whole thing was just one little rumor that had been in one newspaper. Lenny had to do it. He set his jaw and went back to his office to make telephone calls, a hussar of the tax shelter Light Brigade charging into the cannons of a terrified investing public.

Lenny sat down on his chair. He might as well have been in a blackened cell as in a fortieth-floor room with sunlight pouring in the windows. In his brain, a roaring voice told him that he must, absolutely must, without any question at all, break through the fears of the buyers, make them start buying again. He had no possible option except to succeed. He was a man facing a firing squad the next morning if he did not succeed this afternoon. If he could not make a florist from Pasadena get in on a deal, he would be a dead man. If he could not talk an heiress from Brentwood Park into anteing up, he might as well be torn to pieces by wild hyenas.

For two hours, Lenny called as fast as his fingers could dial. He called the people in small towns, the ones who might not have read today's *Wall Street Journal*. He called drilling-rig proprietors in Oroville, grocery-store owners in Bakersfield, almond growers in Sacramento. He put in his best pitches. He sold like he had never sold in his life.

"How are you, Dr. Yamamoto?" Lenny asked. "I'm sorry to call you so late. I don't want to put any pressure on you at all and I probably shouldn't even be doing this, but I just wanted to tell you that we have a chance just for this week to take in a few more partners in the La Cienega project. That's the one where we've already been offered twice as much for the land as we paid for it. It's a real fluke. There's a profit going in. I thought since you had been such a good friend when I was up in Sacramento that I would see if you were interested. Absolutely no pressure on this, doctor. There's a waiting list out the door if you're not interested."

Lenny clenched his fists so tightly that his fingernails made his palms bleed as he talked.

Dr. Yamamoto said that he was really sorry but that he was going to expand his almond groves this year instead and thanks anyway. The underground-communications net of tax avoiders had spread so fast that even Lenny's flying dialing fingers, even his ingenuity, even his persistence, even his virtuosity of sales, could not catch up. No one wanted to end up in tax court.

And still Lenny called. Everyone else at Century West Equities had gone home, and still Lenny called. He had had the foresight to take the home numbers of his clients. Now, as the dental surgeons, clock-shop owners, sportswear manufacturers, credit plumbers, TV talk-show hosts, and lawyers returned home at the end of the day, their wives handed them the telephone and told them that Lenny Brown was on the line. Lenny could hear the squeaking noise as the husbands put their palms over the mouthpiece of the receiver and told the wives to say that they were not home.

"I'm awfully sorry," the wives would say brightly. "But Rick isn't back yet. That was Teddy, our son."

From his window, Lenny saw the sun sinking off toward Malibu. Would he never be able to rent a cottage in the colony again? Would he just go to public beaches like the old failure Lenny Brown? He was getting light-headed from concentrating so hard. His fingers trembled as he dialed. He reached the fifteenth man he called. The man was a personal-injury lawyer in Studio City, a plainspoken guy named Bob. Bob listened carefully to Lenny's pitch, which was the best pitch Lenny had ever given. It was soft-sell, filled with statistics, references to various IRC regs, and inquiries after the health of Bob's wife and children. At the end of it, Bob cleared his throat and said, "Lenny, you're not going to pee one drop after the story in today's *Wall Street Journal*. You come back to me when the whole thing's straightened out, and maybe we can make a deal."

"Bob," Lenny said, "the whole thing in the *Journal* is just a rumor. Anyway, even without the tax angle, it's a very sweet deal."

"Lenny," Bob said. "Call me when the *Journal* has another story saying that the first article was wrong. I gotta go now," he added. "I have to play a set of tennis before dinner or I feel like a fire hydrant."

It was eight o'clock. Lenny could feel cotton growing inside his mouth. He saw red spots in front of his eyes. He remembered that he and Linda were supposed to go over to a party at Joel's by nine.

Like a fighter dragging himself off the canvas after the crowd has left, Lenny scraped himself out of his office and headed for the elevator. Only one elevator was running. Lenny rode it all forty floors down, all by himself. As he fell downward to the ground of West Los Angeles, Lenny thought he was going to collapse on the floor of the elevator. He put his hands on the railing to steady himself. Once he had seen a movie about a radio star who makes a terrible mistake on the air. He leaves in an elevator to go down. As he descends in the elevator, the studio switchboard lights up with angry calls. By the time the star reaches the ground floor, his career is over. Lenny thought of the story and shook with despair and anger.

It was all so incredibly unfair. He had just really gotten rolling, just started to get the beautiful things of life, the recognition, satisfaction, *money*, that he had always deserved and never really thought he would have. Now it was being snatched away from him. It was so bitter he could taste it.

The man in the parking lot took Lenny's ticket and ran to fetch Lenny's car. Lenny always parked in the valet section. It was a little more expensive, but it was a lot less than having a chauffeur-driven car, which is what Joel had. From now on, Lenny thought, he would have to park in the self-parking section. He could save three dollars a day that way. When the man brought Lenny's car, he touched his forehead in a rough salute. He smiled and held out his hand for the dollar Lenny always gave him. This time, Lenny gave him fifty cents. The man looked so wounded that Lenny gave him another fifty cents. (That act alone revealed a sensitivity which by itself doomed Lenny in Los Angeles, as I now understand.)

In the car, Lenny turned the radio to one station after another. He finally settled on a classical station that was playing a well-known processional whose name Lenny could not recall. The car would probably have to go soon, too. Everything would go, if Lenny could not somehow overcome the panic which had gripped his clients. It was just imperative that Lenny, by himself, by his own Brooklyn-born self, crash through the wall of resistance which had been set up by the largest newspaper in America and the Treasury Department of the United States. It was so unfair that Lenny had to take on such an uneven struggle that Lenny could hardly breathe. On Santa Monica Boulevard, right in front of the Beverly Hilton Hotel, Lenny thought he might have to pull over or something. He could not catch his breath. Cars started to honk at him. Finally, he did catch his breath and continued on his way home.

He drove past the magnificent lawns of Beverly Hills. It had been hard enough when he was poor, when he was just a schmuck pulling his putz back in New York. It had been wonderful when he had skyrocketed upward. But it would be unbearable if suddenly he were to have to give up all his hopes, his plans, his certainties about where he would live. To have tasted the life of private planes and Mercedes convertibles and tables in the front room at La Scala and suites at the Princess Hotel; to have promised it to his wife for all time, and then to have to go back to dodging bill collectors and traveling in tour groups and eating Hamburger Helper—it was so painful it made Lenny wish he were dead.

Really, it would be better if Lenny were dead. He would be a laughingstock, a schmuck, a guy who had gone soft when he needed to be hard. It would be bad enough in front of Joel and Michael and Rochelle. That would be torture. But to have to look at himself in the mirror every morning and know that there were two Lenny's, the schmuck Lenny and the successful Lenny and that the successful Lenny was the phony and the schmuck Lenny was real, to know that truth would be fucking unlivable.

It wasn't even really the money or the cars or the plane. That was just window dressing. The lethal loss was that feeling Lenny had once had that he was going places, that he had a future, that he had come into his own, that the perpetual struggle was over. Now he would be back where he had always been, struggling, hustling, scuffling, just another vacuum-cleaner salesman going door to door. Ashes smothered Lenny's heart.

As he pulled up La Cienega toward Sunset Boulevard, he began to calculate how much money he owed. He felt as if an icy hand had grasped his spine. At Flippers, the roller skaters did tight circles in their skintight shorts while the motorists slowed to stare at them. Inside Lenny's car, stopped in the traffic, he realized that he was staring at a major catastrophe. He had taken every penny he had in the bank, plus a loan of fifty-seven thousand dollars, to give Joel a check for a hundred thousand to put down on the discotheque in Cabo San Lucas. He had borrowed the ten thousand down payment on Linda's ballet studio. He had an American Express bill coming in which was going to run at least six thousand dollars. He was supposed to pay the rest of the money for the ballet studio within ten days. That came to a hundred seventy-seven thousand dollars. He was supposed to come up with another hundred thousand for Joel and the disco within sixty days. He had maybe six or seven thousand in his checking account, and that would be gone in a flash.

As Lenny turned onto Sunset, he saw himself as a mountain climber who sees a rat gnawing on the rope that holds him to the side of the mountain and to life. The rope was very nearly gone. Lenny began to sweat. Max was not only not going to give out any more paychecks. He wanted Lenny to start paying rent on the house, the lease on the Mercedes, part of the overhead at the office.

Jesus, Lenny thought. His mouth went dry as his palms sweated onto the steering wheel.

It was goddam easy for Max to say that there wouldn't be any money coming in. He had money in the bank. He could probably live for a thousand years on the interest alone. Max was already there. He hadn't had to extend himself and take a chance for a long time now. Max wouldn't be caught short, owing two hundred thousand bucks without a penny coming in. Max thought too small ever to get himself into a position like that. But people like Lenny who thought big, who had to play catch-up ball, who had to take risks to be the people they were destined to be—those people who really made the big deals happen—got caught like a drowning rat. It was not just cruel. It was outrageous for Max to be so fucking calm about it. Max could spend six years playing golf at the Riviera Country Club, and Shelly Sherman would not miss a single trip to Elizabeth Arden.

And that was it. That was the whole fucking thing. It was not just that Lenny was caught in the swamp with the alligators closing in on his balls. If necessary, Lenny could always just disappear and sell Xerox toner in Oklahoma City. But for Linda it would be even harder. She had been promised that her days as a drone were over. She had stood by Lenny during all the bad years when they had to worry about paying Master Charge every month and had to take the subway. She had stayed with Lenny and never, not ever, come even close to complaining. She had been born again as a happy child when they came to Los Angeles. Lenny had seen her without her brow furrowed. Now was he going to have to tell her that everything would be back the same as it had been (only far worse), with her typing in a typing pool and having to worry about whether or not they could afford new tires for the Toyota?

Lenny walked into the house. It was all dark. Linda was apparently out at her ballet class. Daisy, the black cocker spaniel, ran out of the bedroom and leaped up at Lenny's knees. Daisy, he thought, you are the absolutely only one in the whole world who doesn't know and doesn't care. He picked up Daisy and let her kiss his face. That was love. He put her down and led her into the kitchen. From a huge ceramic mouse he drew a Milk-Bone and handed it to Daisy. She held it in her mouth, wagged her tail, then scampered off into the bedroom. She liked to eat her dog biscuits in private.

Daisy knew nothing about investment tax credits, limited partnerships, nonrecourse notes, investor confidence, Gulfstream II's, no-limit at Caesar's baccarat table, partnerships in discotheques in Cabo San Lucas. What was more, Daisy knew nothing about success or failure, struggle and rest. For Daisy, life was breakfast in the morning and then sleep for the rest of the day. Pet dogs knew absolutely nothing about the whole concept of being in constant turmoil and agony, glimpsing paradise, and then receding into a deeper level of hell than Lenny had even dreamed of back in Brooklyn or Manhattan.

Once, when Lenny had first moved to Los Angeles, he had looked at property on Mulholland Drive, the semirustic highway that runs along the mountains that divide Los Angeles in two. It was about ten A.M. There were no cars except Lenny's. It was a sensationally hot day. Along the road, by brown brush and broken glass, ran a large collie. It had no collar. Its eyes were crazed with fear. Its mouth was open in a crying, drooling pant. Lenny slowed down his car and tried to make the collie get in. He thought he would calm the collie down, then give it to Linda. But the collie would not come near its rescuer. Instead, it ran even faster when Lenny came near. Every time Lenny tried to catch the collie, it looked terrified, then ran away. It was emaciated and had sores on its face. Lenny tried to save it for half an hour. Finally it ran down into a brushy ravine. The collie was simply too berserk at being lost and abandoned to let anyone come near it to rescue it. Lenny drove on to the building site, but forever after, he remembered the lost dog on the Mulholland highway, out of its mind with fear, too maddened with terror to be saved.

That was how Lenny felt, sitting in his living room, waiting for Linda to come home. He did not turn on any lights. He simply sat in the dark and watched the lights of Los Angeles. He was absolutely maddened with fear and desperation. The shark was very near his heart at that moment.

When Lenny had been home for about fifteen minutes, Daisy came out of the bedroom and jumped up on the couch next to him. She walked around in a circle, then collapsed so that she was lying next to Lenny. He stroked her head and said nothing. Lenny loved animals beyond my poor power of description.

At about nine P.M., Linda came home. As soon as she saw that Lenny's car was there and that the lights were out, she knew something was wrong. Once before, three years earlier, she had appeared in their apartment to find Lenny sitting in the dark. That was the day he was fired from a venture-capital firm because he had told off one of the partners for treating him like a servant. Now the lights were out at the house in the Hollywood Hills, and something terrible had happened. She was wearing a pink ballet outfit and Sasson jeans. Her hair was in a chignon. She felt humiliated at that exact moment to be wearing the clothes of play, the clothes of a carefree child, when Lenny was in so much pain. Still, she squared her shoulders, took her groceries out of the car, and walked into the house.

Lenny did not get up. Linda put the groceries down on the flagstone floor of the entryway. She walked over to the couch and sat down next to Lenny. She took his hand. It was exceptionally warm. She kissed him on the cheek. "How are you, Lenny?" she asked in a soft voice.

"Fine," Lenny said. "Just fine." He really did not even know where to begin. How do you begin to climb out of hell?

Linda placed her outstretched palm on Lenny's neck and pulled his face to hers. She kissed him lightly on the lips. "Whatever it is, Lenny," she said, "no matter what it is, we'll be all right. I don't care what happened. I still love you and you're my husband and it'll all be all right. No matter what it is, we'll do all right. I'll sell my car and we'll get a little apartment somewhere that takes dogs and I'll go back to work as a secretary. I can still type real fast. I'm not rusty at all. Really, I'd like to go back to work. It's boring not doing anything all day."

Lenny held his hands up to his eyes, as if his head would fall off his body if he did not support it. "It's been boring?" he asked. "Boring? I've been breaking my balls out there so you wouldn't have to work, and it's been boring?"

Linda could tell Lenny was really upset. He started fights so rarely she could hardly remember the last time.

"I didn't mean it was boring, Lenny," Linda said. "I just meant that I'd like to go back to work. I've had a wonderful time here, but that's not all there is to life. I'd like to go back to work."

"I just put ten thousand dollars down on a ballet studio for you, and you want to go back to typing?" Lenny demanded.

"We'll get that money back," Linda said. "I was never really good enough to have my own ballet studio, anyway. That was just a really silly idea I had. It was crazy. I'll talk to that Hungarian guy and get our money back."

Lenny abruptly stood up and walked up and down the length of the living room. "We can't get the money back. It was nonrefundable. It said that in the contract. If you didn't want to have a studio, why did I throw out that money?"

"I don't know," Linda said. "It was really crazy of me. Really, really crazy. I know I can get that man to give us the money back. I just know it. Please come and sit down next to me and tell me what happened."

"You think that crook is going to give us back our deposit?" Lenny asked in a hiss. "No fucking way. That money is totally and completely gone. Completely." Lenny glanced over at the porcelain-finish Cartier clock on the end table next to the couch. It cost three hundred dollars. One day Lenny had bought four of them and scattered them around the house for Linda because she liked things that were cute and old-fashioned like Cartier clocks. He suddenly stood up and grasped the clock. He threw it against the wall. It smashed into shards of glass and brass gears. Lenny sank back onto the couch. Neither Linda nor the dog made a sound. "You never noticed them after the first day I bought them, anyway," Lenny said. "So what does it matter if I at least get a little enjoyment out of them?"

Linda looked out the window at the hundreds of thousands of people who were going about their daily lives without suffering devastating blows of low self-esteem, anxiety, and terror. Out that window, in greater Los Angeles, there had to be people who ran out to Thrifty Drugs for a pack of cigarettes and did not feel as if their world was collapsing in upon them. There had to be people who lived a quiet life at Lockheed or P. G. & E. and came home to eat a simple meal and did not feel utterly lost. Linda thought that, and then she took Lenny's hand again. "I know that we can get that money back for the ballet studio," she said. "And I just know that Joel can give you back the money for the disco in Cabo San Lucas. He said there were a million people waiting to invest, so why should he care whether he gets the money from you or someone else?"

"Everybody always says he can get the money from anyone," Lenny said. "That's part of the game."

"What happened?" Linda asked. "Did you have a fight with Max?"

Lenny shook his head. He let out a long sigh. "I wish that's all it was," he said. "Max and I are in great shape. It's not Max. It's me. I have totally and completely wrecked everything."

"Lenny, whatever it is, it'll pass," Linda said. "In a year, we won't even think about it. In two years, we won't be able to remember it even if we try."

Lenny laughed bitterly. "If all's well, in a year I'll be dead and you'll have a husband who doesn't wreck everyone's life."

Linda put her hand on Lenny's neck and stroked it gently. She leaned forward and kissed him on the cheek. "I promise you, Lenny, whatever it is, it'll be all right."

"The hell it will," Lenny said. Then he put his face in his hands and closed his eyes. Linda stroked his back and put her cheek against his shoulder. Lenny sat up after a minute and said, "All right, I'll explain it to you, and I won't blame you at all if you leave and don't ever come back. There's no reason someone like you should be stuck with someone like me. I'm just too much of a failure for someone like you."

"Stop it, Lenny," Linda said softly. "Just stop it and let me help you."

Then Lenny told Linda about how they were in hock a hundred feet above their heads and how there was no way on earth that they were going to get out of hock anytime, because now Lenny had lost any hope of making any real money for six months at least and maybe a year. Meanwhile, Lenny owed money to everyone you could think of for ballet studios and discotheques in Cabo San Lucas. He also owed a lot on his airplane and on his American Express and on his Diner's Club and Master Charge and Visa, for that matter.

"And all from one fucking article in the *Wall Street Journal* that probably isn't true, anyway," he added. "This whole way we live, the whole fucking way, it's all based on money coming in. I thought money would be coming in forever. It was so fucking easy, and then it all came to nothing. I was just completely crazy. I got us into such deep craziness that we're never ever gonna get out."

"Lenny," Linda said, "money troubles are not the worst kind of troubles to have. So we don't pay these people. So what? It's not the end of the world. People don't pay other people all the time. It happens all the time. Even if we have to go bankrupt, so what? They can't take us away from each other. They can't take Daisy away."

Linda kissed Lenny on the cheek, but he shook her away irritably. Somehow, after all their years together, she still could not fully plumb Lenny's depths of despair and self-hate. Of course, the money was not the real problem. No one in America starves. The problem was that the money was a way of keeping score, and now Lenny had lost the game. It was not disappointing the Hungarian or the disco people or even American Express cards that was the problem. The problem was that Lenny *and everyone else* could now see that Lenny was a complete schmuck, the kind of asshole who put on a big show but couldn't cut the mustard when the time came for mustard cutting. The problem was that Lenny thought he had left misery and failure behind, and now they had sprung back on him bigger and stronger than ever.

Lenny started to pace back and forth in the living room. He held his hands to his head as if it might fall off without help and support from the rest of his body.

Linda had never felt that her right to life and breath depended upon how much money she made or how much she accomplished or how successful her friends thought she was. She had an idea that she was an ordinary person who, by virtue of continuing to be alive, deserved to continue in that state. She could not exactly understand how badly Lenny felt, just as a person who is sighted cannot ever understand fully how a blind person feels. She could see that Lenny was suffering, though (this part of the story is almost all from her recollections of the night and what Lenny told her), and she was determined to do something about it.

"Listen," she said, "how can you be sure that the business will be closed down for six months?"

Lenny waved at her as if she had just said something preposterous. "Max said it, and I think Max knows pretty well about these things. A goddam sight better than I do, that's for sure."

"Listen," Linda said. "Assuming, just assuming that your business is closed down for six months, tell me this. Why can't you work for someone else?"

Lenny looked at her pityingly. "The whole real-estate scam is closed down," he said. "Nobody's doing any business."

Linda stood up and walked over to Lenny to comfort him. She grasped his arm just above the elbow and stared right into his eyes. "Lenny," she said, "I don't really care if we're poor. And I don't mind going back to work. I never cared whether I was rich or poor. I just wanted you. But if you're really that fantastically dead set on making money, why can't you sell something else? You're a fantastic salesman. You're the best salesman in the world. Why can't you sell something else? Why can't you sell computers or airplanes or something else? There must be a lot of money in them."

Lenny stopped in his tracks. "I can't just change overnight," he said. "I don't know anything about planes or computers. You have to know something about those things to be able to sell them." Still, his voice was different. He was thinking about Linda's suggestion. Actually, it was a possibility. He was a helluva salesman.

"I know you can sell anything," Linda said. "You've told me a million times that it isn't knowing about the product that sells, it's knowing about people."

"What're we going to do while I'm learning how to sell something else?" Lenny asked. "What about the name I've got in this business? Am I supposed to throw that all away?"

"Lenny, what does General Motors do when it can't pay its bills right away? The guys wait. They've gotten used to it. And I'll bet every sales organization in L.A. knows how you can sell. That kind of reputation doesn't just stay in real estate. After all, people who had nothing to do with the circus knew all about P. T. Barnum, and you're better than P. T. Barnum."

"Much better," Lenny said, and then he laughed. Then he hugged Linda and said, "If I ever get any money again, I'm gonna build a statue to you right in that park in Beverly Hills. To my wife, who saved my life."

Lenny was still pale and ashen. The shark was still circling hungrily around his heart. But now Lenny knew that at least he had a chance. The sky was no longer completely leaden. Out in the far west, toward Hawaii, there was still a faint light.

Lenny talked about what kind of salesman he might be. He had read in the *Wall Street Journal* that people were selling freight-car-ownership tax shelters. That was a possibility, since it was a related field. He might also want to get into computers, since they were becoming bigger all the time. In the future, every family would have a computer, and he wanted to be in on it. Linda reminded Lenny about Joel's party. Lenny said that he had better invite Ben Stein along, since Ben Stein was really wired in a lot of different areas and could probably give him a lot of pointers about where he should go next. Still, when Lenny dialed the telephone to call me, his fingers shook. Linda remembered that. She remembered every detail of that evening since it was the beginning of the end of Lenny, and even now she still loves him.

THE RIVER

There was heavy traffic on Sunset Boulevard that night. I remember because Lenny had time to explain everything that had happened, about the *Wall Street Journal*, about the telephone calls to doctors and dentists, about how much money he owed (he laughed when he talked about the disco and the Hungarian, but it was a hollow laugh). Lenny also had time to get into a swearing contest with a car full of Mexicans that kept veering into our lane. His face became red as he talked about hundred-thousand-dollar notes coming due and shit-eating beaners in a shit-eating Camaro all in the same breath.

"If I can just restructure all my debts, get a little breathing space, maybe offer to up the interest a little . . . look at those assholes, hey, assholes, get out of the road . . . and then maybe try to get something started in time sharing on computers or maybe freight-car shelters which are supposed to be extremely big these days or maybe even in airplanes which have to be gigantic because look how much one 747 has to cost . . ."

Still, Lenny's temples were damp with perspiration even though the air-conditioning in my car was going full blast. His voice cracked when he talked about trying to persuade the bank to give him more time to pay back his note. I told him what I knew about the other fields, which wasn't much, and that a good salesman like Lenny should have no trouble making a lot of money in airplanes or computers or chemicals. ("Chemicals!" Lenny said. "Tell me about chemicals!") Then we were at the party.

In front of the house were the usual black Porsches, black Mercedes, black Rolls sedans, even a black Rolls convertible or two. Lights glittered inside the windows. In the living room, two servants in black uniforms passed out drinks and canapés. I noticed that Lenny had two scotch and waters before he even said hello to anyone. Linda looked at him closely. Joel came up to Lenny, looking more like a Yeshiva *bucher* than ever. He wrapped his arm around Lenny's shoulder and led him off. As he did, I could hear him say, "Listen, the situation in Cabo San Lucas is looking even better than I thought it would. We can probably get started much sooner than I thought if we can get the money together." Even from behind, I could see Lenny slouch with discouragement. Then they disappeared from the room out to the swimming pool.

Rochelle appeared out of nowhere. She wore tight jeans and a T-shirt that said "Cataclysmic Variables" and then gave the date and place of a conference on astrophysics. Her little features looked unusually relaxed. She talked to me and Linda for a few minutes in a slurred voice. "I really can't believe Joel," she said. "I told him I wanted to bring my parents out here and that I couldn't do it on my stewardess pass, so he says he'll get me tickets. He gets me fucking SuperSavers, like my parents are supposed to come visit their daughter and her millionaire boyfriend and they're sitting in the back with the high school kids on a fucking field trip. What a putz. I really can't believe him. A complete and total schmuck. Complete and total." It took Rochelle about five minutes to say that, and then she staggered off toward the pool. Linda and I sat down and talked about what we could do to get Lenny back onto the track of self-esteem, which in his case was the same as the track of staying alive. We talked about jobs he might get and things we might tell him that would cheer him up. I had the idea of offering him to my pal, the powerful TV producer, to see if the powerful TV producer cared to hire him as a salesman of syndicated TV shows. Linda and I convinced ourselves that Lenny would be all right. In the meantime, Lenny was talking to Joel and would not be all right.

Joel took Lenny off to the pool house, a spacious two-story affair with wicker furniture and terra cotta tile floors leading to magnificently white French doors. There were a few other people sitting in the pool house, sniffing up cocaine from the glass top of a coffee table. Two women and a man sat silently, occasionally bending over the table to take in the drug through a silver straw. They paid no attention to Joel and Lenny. Every few minutes one of them would throw back his head and say, "Ha-cha-cha," and then laugh.

Joel told Lenny that the main hotel in Cabo San Lucas had so many advance bookings that it would probably open two months early. In fact, it had so many bookings that the owners were already starting work on a new wing that they had not planned to begin until 1980. "You know who's making these reservations?" Joel asked. "Young single people from L.A. and Chicago and Dallas and Houston and Cleveland. Kids with money in their pockets and sex on their minds. So where should they want to go but to our disco when they get to town? That's where the action is. Not on the fucking beach."

Lenny did not say anything. He began to hyperventilate.

"Those kids don't know how much a fucking peso is worth. We can charge five bucks for a glass of white wine, and they won't even know. But we've got to get the decorators in there right away. And I think we've really got to take the cork out about decorating. We want people from Shaker Heights to go back home and say there's the most beautiful discotheque in the world there in some fucking little town in Mexico," Joel said. "When people are really drunk and nervous, they like to be in a fancy room. That's a fact of life," Joel added.

Lenny said, "I don't know, Joel. I really don't know."

"What don't you know, pal?" Joel asked. "The numbers don't look right to you anymore?"

Lenny wiped his forehead. "It's not exactly that," he said. "Not that at all."

Joel slapped Lenny on the back. "Are you worried about that business in the *Wall Street Journal* today?" he asked. "I talked to Max. He says things are going to be slow for a while. So what? With the money you've been making, you can ride out the wait. A guy with a balance sheet like yours, a guy who can sell like you, shouldn't have any trouble. Listen, I know sometimes you really hate to take money out of those CD's to buy into something risky like a disco, but I think you could get by with just a few hundred thousand in the bank and put the rest into some big-money projects."

Lenny smiled weakly. At that moment he had about six thousand dollars in the bank and debts of about fifty times that much. The idea of living on the mythical fortune he supposedly had stashed away was both hysterically funny and hysterically terrifying.

"I don't know," Lenny said. "I have a lot of obligations, and it's going to be a pretty dry period over at Century West Equities." He tried, by his colloquial speech and relaxed syntax, to hide a tingling feeling that was growing at the base of his spine. By talking slowly, he tried to conceal an anxiety which was building inside him like a volcano in eruption. The sense of possibility he had felt when Linda and I reassured him in the car was rapidly fading. It was being replaced by the feeling that he had been a fool yet again to allow himself to be calmed. Of course he was in desperate trouble. There was no time to learn about computers or freight cars. The crisis was critical right this very moment. Joel and the Hungarian and American Express needed the money this very instant, not after he had learned the ropes at Honeywell or Boeing. He could not get by being a little late with his credit-card payments. He had been playing with the big boys with big bucks. And he had got caught with his pants down. In a way, he was already fucked. After all, even if Joel didn't know, Joel would know, and anyway, Lenny knew. He was going to default before everyone who counted.

In the pool house, he started to sweat. His fingers shook. He reached into a crystal bowl for a cigarette. Joel had thoughtfully set out Philip Morris cigarettes for all his guests. Joel had never seen Lenny smoke or shake or sweat indoors. He was concerned. Above the noise of the stereo ("Sergeant Pepper's Loney Hearts' Club Band"), Joel spoke to Lenny.

"Listen, boychik," he said, "I've been in business a little bit longer than you. Lemme tell you something. You're not the first person who feels as if the bottom just fell out. It happens to everyone in business a few times a year. That's business. If you're into thinking that it's the worst thing that's ever happened, forget it. That's never the way it is. I don't care if you're broke or bankrupt or anything. A guy like you will get over it."

Lenny looked at Joel with tears in his eyes. Joel was so good, so understanding, so generous of spirit to see clearly into Lenny's troubled heart and offer solace. Lenny actually felt better. Just hearing Joel say those things made Lenny feel better. After all, Joel was a man of the world. Still, Lenny felt a tingling in his spine.

Joel touched Lenny's knee and added, "Listen, pal, I can see you're still a little upset. I'll tell you what I do when a bank calls and tells me they can't lend me the money I've already spent."

"Oh, it's not that bad," Lenny lied. But his palms were sweating.

"Listen, God made some scientists so smart that they invented these pills, Lenny," Joel said. He opened his palm. On it were lying eight large round white pills. Some of them were scored in the middle. Others said "Rorer" and then some numbers that Lenny could not read. "Take a couple of these, and you'll really feel as if you didn't give a damn about anything. Really. They just take away the pain for a while. They make you feel as if you were out on a cloud somewhere."

"I don't take any drugs," Lenny said. "It keeps me out of trouble." Still, his fingers shook and his face was becoming pale.

"Go ahead," Joel said, "I take them all the time. If you don't take them yet, you're the last one in town. Go ahead." He handed Lenny a glass of scotch and two pills. "Take either one or two. If you get sick from it, I'll give you my car."

Lenny laughed and reached for two of the pills. He swallowed them and then chased them with scotch (Johnny Walker Black).

"At least they don't crumble up and taste bitter like aspirin," Lenny said. "How long until they hit me?"

"It all depends," Joel said. "And don't expect to get high like with marijuana. You just feel real relaxed."

"What are they?" Lenny said. "Jesus, I must be losing my mind. I didn't even ask you what they were." He shook his head and sweated still more. Christ, he thought, I am really cracking up. Who takes drugs without even knowing what they are? Crazy people. Losers.

"They're Quaaludes," Joel said. "Strictly from the factory. No bootlegs from Mexico or somewhere."

"What are Quaaludes?" Lenny asked. "I've read about them, but I can't think what they are. Sleeping pills?"

"They're sort of like sleeping pills," Joel said, "except that they make you feel absolutely great if you fight going to sleep. You'll feel a little drowsy, and then you'll feel great."

For an instant, Joel thought that Lenny might pass out. That was how worried he looked. He was not even looking at the incredible girl in the disco pants and the black T-shirt who was dancing by herself in the pool house. Joel thought it would be better to leave Lenny alone for a few minutes. Take off the pressure to talk. Joel got up to talk to the girl in the maroon disco pants. Her name was Caryn, with a C, and she was in car leasing.

For the first time that day, Lenny thought about nothing. He was so petrified of his failure, and now of his possible self-poisoning, that his sensory synapses were temporarily overwhelmed and silent. He looked about the room at the girls in skintight jeans, in T-shirts or tube tops, with pale skin and blood-red lipstick, absent but vicious looks about the eyes and a promising, seductive look about the hips and thighs, wrapped in blue denim and bursting with demonic hunger.

He looked at the men in the room. They looked as if they might at any moment be visited by their mothers, who would tell them what good boys they had been for making so much money and making their mothers proud of them at the bridge club in Sarasota. They wore tight jeans, too, and open-necked shirts, no matter how fat they were. As if to confirm an Easterner's satiric vision of Los Angeles, the men wore gold chains with an almost pitiful defiance of what they must have known was good sense. In ten minutes of staring at the people in Joel's pool house, only one thought repeatedly came into Lenny's mind and then disappeared into the void of terror and self-hate which was his soul at that moment. The one thought which came and went, leaving misery in its train, was only this: How the hell can all these people make money and get along all right in life when I can't? What's wrong with me?

But that thought ravaged Lenny's spirit for only ten minutes, because after ten minutes, Lenny started to feel a tingling in his fingers and his toes. It was unusual because, although it should have been worrisome, it was pleasant. Lenny felt like giggling. He looked at the room. It was superficially the same, except that he no longer felt any envy or animosity toward the men and women in their tight jeans. A minute ago he had totally had it in for them. Now, they were all brothers and sisters. He almost stood up and started to hug the men and women. But when he began to get up, he felt phenomenally tired, in a delicious, dreamy kind of way. He sat back down and laughed out loud. These people in the pool house were fine people, the kind of people you could trust with your life. The girls were sexually exciting but friendly. The air in the room, which had seemed hot and damp, now seemed tropical and balmy. Lenny felt tired again, but not as if he wanted to sleep. He felt tired as in *relaxed* completely.

Lenny had smoked marijuana before. Five or six times back in college, he and Linda had toked up on a J, then strolled around Washington Square. He remembered the hallucinations, the passersby coming in and out of focus, the lapses of memory, the whirling street lamps and sidewalks. He could feel the Beatles' lyrics in his blood in those days. Marijuana was a wild, confusing aura closing over the brain. Lenny stopped doing it because it made him feel anxious. He had a hard enough time assimilating the reality of his struggle. To add another layer of the semi-real was intolerable.

Tonight in the pool house was different. The Quaaludes washed away from Lenny every gram of the weight of anxiety which had been pressing upon his mind. As the drug dissolved and flowed through his bloodstream, Lenny felt as if he had been bathed in forgiveness. There was no longer any doubt about how wonderful life was. There were no demands, no necessity of accomplishing anything. The Hungarian and the discotheque and Century West Equities were a million miles away in an unapproachable pit, while Lenny floated in a warm, caressing sea of complete acceptance.

Lenny slouched upon the couch and smiled. He closed his eyes. The room did not spin. Instead, he felt as if a wave of heaven's mercy were carrying him ever higher into a new dimension of peace. Yes, that was exactly it. Lenny, who had never known a moment of waking peace for as long as he could remember, now sailed in a perfectly azure sky, far away from the hell which had so permanently raged inside him.

Joel finished making a firm rendezvous with Caryn for the next day at her apartment in North Hollywood, then looked over to see a transformed Lenny. He sat down next to Lenny just as Lenny was rubbing his cheeks, realizing that they were numb. "Joel, my pal," Lenny said. "This is really a great party."

Joel was happy to see Lenny in a better state of mind. He took Lenny's hand away from his cheek and opened it. In the palm of Lenny's hand, Joel laid ten Quaaludes. "Now listen, Lenny," he said. "You give a couple of these to Linda and then don't take any more until you get home. Then take some and get into the jacuzzi."

"You're a pal, Joel," Lenny said. "A pal."

Lenny staggered out of the pool house. He looked at a girl swimming in the pool in a black maillot cut up to her waist. She looked spectral, unreal, in a perfect blue gem set in Lenny's backyard. Lenny was not hallucinating. He simply felt so good that he was thinking in poetic terms.

He found Linda in the sitting room just off the living room, on a white love seat in front of a glass table covered with plates of cheese. He slumped down on the seat next to her and brushed her cheek with his lips. "I don't know how I got so lucky as to have you," he said. "You're the best thing that ever happened to me."

Linda was so overjoyed to see Lenny's mood changed—and obviously not drunk, since Lenny *never* drank too much—that her eyes grew moist. She squeezed Lenny's hand in the code they had used on the plane coming out from New York two years before. *I love you.* Lenny squeezed back, *How much?* Linda answered, *A lot.* Then Linda leaned her head on Lenny's shoulder and told him she knew everything would be all right.

"I know it will," Lenny said. "I want you to take one of these," he added, holding out a Quaalude. He already had enough sense to put the rest of them in a pocket. "They're not a narcotic. They're a sleeping pill and they feel great."

I know that in most stories, the villain has to persuade the victim to take the drug, to break down resistance to a vicious habit such as taking hypnotics or opiates. But since I was in the room, I can tell you that in Linda's case, it did not happen that way. Linda trusted Lenny so completely, felt so badly, wanted to feel better so desperately, wanted to show Lenny she obeyed him so completely, that she simply said, "What is it?"

Anyway, Lenny was not a villain, and Linda was not a victim.

Lenny said, "It's a Quaalude. A sleeping pill, only it doesn't make you feel sleepy, really. It just makes you feel like goofy or that nothing's wrong."

Linda nodded and looked at me. "That sounds right to me," she said. "Anyway, Benjy's driving." She picked up a vodka Gibson from the coffee table and chased down the 'lude. She swallowed and smiled and said, "It's fine so far."

We talked for about ten minutes, and I noticed that soon both Lenny and Linda's speech was slurred. Linda smiled as broadly as Lenny. She giggled. She rubbed her cheeks. She threw back her head and laughed. She hugged Lenny. She looked as if the tension of the evening had been shed the way a snake sheds its skin.

Her cheeks glowed with red excitement and warmth. Then they turned white and cool to the touch (I touched them). Her eyes were first exceptionally clear and animated, then became glassy and slow-moving.

When she and Lenny talked, they talked in fragments of sentences, always of recollection and nostalgia: "Remember when we took the bus in the snowstorm . . . That guy who sat in front of us in English Lit. with the blue . . . God, I can't believe that girl who used to sell sandwiches . . . Washington Square . . . The snow under the street lights . . . Wow, are we lucky we're not still in that house in SoHo with that old lady . . ." They talked in a language of euphoria and shared memories which were, of course, known only to them. They laughed and laughed as if an angel of the Lord had appeared to them, touched them with a flaming sword, and told them that they would live forever. Although I knew they were happy because of the drug, I was nevertheless glad to see their joy. When I had picked them up perhaps one hour earlier, they looked as crushed as if their lives were destined to be spent under ashes and torment. Now, I thought, the drug will show them that life goes on and that they still had a great many mornings to look forward to. They sat on the love seat, laughing and smiling, and I thought that there was still hope of redemption in this world.

IN THE LAND OF NOD

When you get on the wrong train, every stop is the wrong stop. I drove Lenny and Linda home from the party at about midnight. They sat in the front seat hugging and kissing. We glided through dense traffic on Sunset, but Lenny did not shout at Mexicans. Instead, he smiled and grinned and put his hand under Linda's blouse and kissed her for ten minutes straight. I listened to the "Elvis Hour" on KRLA. When I dropped off Lenny and Linda in front of the house on Hollywood Boulevard I could hear Daisy barking with excitement. She had gotten to know not only the sound of Lenny's car and Linda's car but also the sound of my car. When Lenny got out of the car, under a dazzling California night of blue-black sky and stars, he hugged Linda and turned to me. "Listen, pal, I just want you to know that tonight is something that's never going to happen again," he said.

"What's that?" I asked.

"Being so defeated," he said. "That's not me. I'm not going to go around feeling sorry for myself like that ever again. I'm a very lucky guy."

"Indeed you are," I said.

"I'm just going to be happy now that I've got so much good going on, including good pals like you," he said.

"It's nothing," I said. "Think nothing of it."

But Lenny was already somewhere else, staring blankly at a rose-bush. Linda said good night, and then she and Lenny walked into the house. I did not see them for three days after that. I called over and over again but got a busy signal for three days. I called Lenny at Century West Equities. His secretary said that he was ill and would call me when he returned to work. When he did not return my calls after two days, I went over to the house. It was dark. On the fourth day, he called.

He sounded different, dragged out, silly. As he reconstructed for me what had happened, and as Linda told me later, he and Linda had gone for a long swim in the river Styx.

That first night of Quaaludes, Linda and Lenny had swum in their pool and taken more Quaaludes. They had the irresistible feeling that a new world had been created specifically for them to enjoy. For their whole lives, they had struggled against an invisible screen of anxiety and care. Even Linda, who was far more confident than Lenny, had a million small worries each day about traffic or smog or cleaning or a fingernail or the stack of American Express bills, not to mention the overriding worry about whether her husband would come home from work crazed with frustration and anger. For Lenny, each day (until he came to Los Angeles) had been like running through deep mud. Even in Los Angeles, in the best of times, Lenny had to worry about this strategy or that tactic to sell a syndication, about the straightness of accounting for commissions, about whether Max might start hating him, about whether Joel would become so rich that Lenny could never catch up. Daily life was daily slogging through swamps with heavy packs. Suddenly, with the Quaaludes, Lenny and Linda were lighter than air, frolicking and jumping *against no resistance*. Where had this feeling been all their lives?

Imagine astronauts who have landed on the moon. They can jump fifty feet even in their space suits. There is no gravity to hold them down. That was Lenny and Linda that first night on Quaaludes. Nothing hurt. There were no cares, no worries. Life for them was effortless and frictionless, *like life in a dream.*

They made love in the pool, with the dog, Daisy, lying by the side, slurping water from the jacuzzi. They floated on their backs, staring up at the night sky. The sat in the jacuzzi and giggled. Inside the house, they drank gallons of orange juice and watched a late movie of *The Last Picture Show*. At the point when Ellen Burstyn says, "If it hadn't of been for Sam the Lion, I guess I would have completely missed it, whatever it is," Lenny and Linda looked at each other dreamily. Whatever it was, they would not miss it.

They fell asleep fifteen seconds after they hit the mattress. Lenny, who meticulously showered and flossed his teeth before sleep most nights, simply passed out in his robe, with the television tuned to a display of the week's movies on the Z channel.

They awakened at almost exactly noon the next day. It was a weekday. As always in Los Angeles, the sun poured through the windows like a tidal wave of light, obliterating everything in its path. Lenny and Linda were still fifty percent stoned. I learned later that Quaaludes' active ingredient, Methaqualone, stays in the bloodstream in significant amounts for seventy-two hours. It stays in the bloodstream in sufficient quantity to induce sleep for twenty-four hours. Alas, it does not stay in the bloodstream long enough to induce euphoria for more than a few hours.

Lenny and Linda dragged themselves out of bed and started the routine of the day. Lenny decided not to bother going to work because he was so tired. Instead, he staggered down to the pool, let Daisy evacuate her bowels on the ivy near the pool, then returned to the upstairs before he remembered that he wanted to take a swim to wake himself up. In the heat of noon, under the pitiless Los Angeles sun, Lenny swam a few short laps. Then he sat in the jacuzzi for ten minutes. The telephone was ringing in the room next to the pool, but Lenny did not answer it. He found that instead of becoming more alert and awake, he felt steadily more tired and more dizzy. Somehow the exercise was just stirring up the chemical in his blood, rather than making him vigorous. Lenny swam a few more laps but felt still more tired, so he got out of the pool.

As Lenny sat at his breakfast table, reading a story in the View section of the *Times* ("Jewish Women Stand Up against Israeli Militarism at Dinner in Beverly Hills"), he realized that he did not feel happy. In fact, he felt extremely unhappy. The full extent of his financial and psychological crisis began to press upon him. His mind was befuddled from the drug so he could not even begin to imagine a way out of his humiliation and his debt. Linda would obviously be no help. She staggered around the kitchen like a drugged white mouse in a maze, banging her head against open cupboard doors, stubbing her toe against chairs that had always been there. No,

Lenny was definitely up a creek without a paddle, and all alone to boot.

His hands started to shake as he drank from his cup of herbal tea. He could not eat more than a bite or two of an English muffin. He felt extremely nauseated. Not only that, but his pulse was racing, even though his mind was swathed in raw cotton. Then he remembered something wonderful, like a starving man who recalls that he has a side of roast beef in his refrigerator. He had taken only five of the Quaaludes last night. That included Linda's share. Now he had five left, and that spelled salvation.

"Why should we feel like this?" he asked Linda. "We haven't done anything wrong." He said that as he offered Linda a 'lude with her morning coffee. Linda, who was also feeling a little bent out of shape, swallowed it without a murmur. Lenny broke one of his 'ludes in half and took it with a whole one. This time something miraculous happened. Lenny and Linda did not even have to wait for the drug to be metabolized by the stomach and the small intestine, did not have to wait for the methaqualone molecules to meet the receptors in their cerebra. Just knowing that they had swallowed salvation was enough to lift them out of their mood almost immediately. If a bankrupt man receives a large check in the mail, he does not have to cash the check to know that he is saved. Neither did the drug have to reach the brain for Lenny and Linda to realize that their future, at least for the next two hours, was assured. The check was in their hands. Not only that, it was a certified check. It had worked last night, so it was bound to work today.

In a few minutes, Linda cleared away the dishes. She wanted everything to be really neat while she was high. Lenny showered again and shaved. The great kindness of the drug showed itself to him when he was in the shower. A perfectly prosaic experience became a work of art, a moment to remember. The cascading water, the warm sheets of wetness, all made possible by great aqueducts and pumping stations and thousands of miles of concrete and oil imported from Indonesia, equipment manned by poor schmucks who were not blissed out on 'ludes, all of these things impressed Lenny.

The warm water penetrated into Lenny's pores at about the moment the 'ludes hit his cortex. Surrounded by deep blue tiles, rising steam, and a few notes of music from his own throat, Lenny sensed the aggravation running out of his body, down his legs, and into the drain, as if he had somehow willed it out of his system. It was a true gift from the gods. He felt so relaxed that he began to giggle.

By the time Lenny dried himself and emerged into the bedroom, he was feeling wonderful. Life was so perfect, so endless, that he wondered how anyone had ever felt anything but great.

Linda had dropped a Waterford crystal flower vase on the floor of the kitchen. She was sweeping up the pieces when she began to giggle. She cut herself on a shard of crystal, and still she giggled. She finished sweeping up, then mopped up her blood, then put on a bandage, and then lay on the bed and laughed for ten minutes without stopping. The telephone rang, and Lenny and Linda both laughed. There was a knock on the door. Daisy barked, but Lenny and Linda kept laughing. They even laughed as they made love. They were God's children, immune from the worry or frustration of mortals.

By the middle of the afternoon, Lenny and Linda were both feeling rough around the edges. They had learned enough to know that more 'ludes were the answer to the problem. They each took another, and soon they were feeling like they wanted to feel.

To make this story full, I would have to tell every detail of the next two days. Alas, I do not know them. I do know that twice during the next forty-eight hours, Lenny called Joel and got more 'ludes sent over by cab. I also know that by the end of the three days, Lenny and Linda were so drugged that they slept for thirty-six straight hours.

I also know that by the end of the period of being drugged and sleeping, Lenny had a completely new priority. He was still concerned about Century West Equities, the Hungarian, and the disco in Cabo San Lucas. He was deeply worried about his failure and his humiliation. Lenny was also interested in getting to know how to be a salesman of airliners or computers. But he wanted 'ludes the way a drowning man wants oxygen.

A new job, a long-term loan, even a reprieve from the *Wall Street Journal* would take time. Lenny had learned quite suddenly that the most certain of rescues could fall through. Besides, he was pissed off. He hadn't done anything wrong that he could see, and the roof had fallen in on him. The best way to stay out of trouble for the time being was to get more 'ludes. Once you had them, there were no slipups, no sudden changes, no unpredictable variables. The 'ludes themselves were sufficient. No other contingency needed to occur for the 'ludes to do their work. The line from acquisition of the drug to nirvana was straight and unbroken. No one could change his mind. No bank could fail to come through. No strange article could appear, queering everything. The 'ludes were a completely circular, self-reinforcing stairway to heaven.

Lenny had always been an inventive and ingenious kind of guy. The 'ludes did not dull that aspect of Lenny's personality as much as put it to its highest and best use. The drug might make him euphoric and sleepy, but it also made him eager to devise ever better ways to get it, but I will tell more about that later.

In the week after Lenny and Linda first began to take Quaaludes for the rapid relief of pain, they started to resume a more usual way of living. They did not stay inside their house indefinitely, getting bedsores from sleeping so much. That is not how Quaalude fanatics live. They had their first crazy three days, then their day and a half of sleep, and then they began to go out like normal people. They walked their dog, shopped at the Alpha Beta on the corner of Fairfax and Santa Monica, brought their dry cleaning in to the Sunset Hills cleaners, had their car washed at the Sunset Plaza Car Wash, went to the movies on Hollywood Boulevard or in Westwood, went to Joel's parties, and generally carried on living.

Linda occasionally went to Florence's dance class. Florence criticized Linda for being slow in her turns and jetés, but gradually Linda learned to struggle against the drug while she was at the studio and dance with a semblance of her former grace and quickness. Florence suspected that Linda was on something, but since she suspected that about many of her students at one time or another, she said nothing.

Lenny went in to Century West Equities a few times a week. Nothing much was going on in sales, but there was still a fair amount of property to manage. After all, Lenny and Max had sold many buildings which needed continuous maintenance. Max had thoughtfully assigned all such work to Century West Maintenance, a wholly owned subsidiary of Century West Equities. This little gold mine continued to produce ore. Lenny persuaded Max to put him in charge of the work in west L.A. For that, Lenny got a small salary, the continued use of the Mercedes convertible, and the ability to write checks to pay for janitorial services, exterminators, cleansers, light bulbs, grass seed, and floor polish. The account was not large, but it was a sign of Max's trust in Lenny that Max allowed him to sign checks on the account. At first, Lenny did not abuse the trust. He charged the account for a few meals he had while he was traveling from building to building, and for his gasoline, and even for a couple of lunches at Ma Maison with Joel. But that was a small set of deviations from the straight and narrow. By and large, Lenny merited Max's trust.

Also, Lenny went to Computer Services Corporation in the airport, to Northrup Aircraft, to Hughes Aircraft, and to Scientific Data Systems in Malibu. He talked to the heads of the sales departments at each company. A few of them had even heard of Lenny from his work at Century West. The man at Hughes said that Hughes could definitely use a sharpshooter like Lenny.

The man wore a large-check polyester jacket and had dandruff on his lapels. He smoked a Tiparillo while he talked to Lenny. His office was next to the loading dock of the helicopter division. The air smelled of diesel exhaust and tobacco smoke. The man had bad breath, perhaps from the half-eaten salami sandwich on his desk. The veins in his nose were broken and blue. The man, whose name was Royall Kennedy, Jr., said, "You're a helluva closer, Lenny, which is what we like in this business. You could do well here. A lot of our top men are pulling down fifty thousand a year selling helicopters all over the fucking place. But this ain't the wild west like the real-estate business, Lenny. We have a training program, and then you work your way up. But once you've gotten a little seniority, you're set. Hughes ain't going anywhere."

Lenny said that working for a prestigious company like Hughes meant a lot to him.

Royall Kennedy, Jr., said that if Lenny could learn that this was a corporation, with a lot of different people who didn't like to have their toes stepped on, he would do just fine. "There's no place here for a guy who thinks he's a superstar, though. This is a team. You play by the rules and don't try to hog the show. If you do that, you can count on a lot of years of a good life. Fully paid health plan, use of a company car, and not just some Pinto but a Thunderbird or a Camaro. It's a good life."

Lenny walked out to the parking lot to his Mercedes convertible with tears streaming down his cheeks. So this was what life was going to be like after Century West Equities. He had earned fifty thousand in some good *weeks* in tax shelters. A Camaro? Oh, Jesus. He popped a 'lude while he was driving home along the freeway. By the time he reached the La Cienega exit, he was sure he could think of something better than Hughes Aircraft.

A new computer company called Differential Intelligence also offered Lenny a job. But for Lenny to start work, he had to learn how to program and access a computer. This was no small job for a man who had taken two 'ludes before his first lesson. Lenny left the lesson after fifteen minutes. He explained to the teacher, a sincere woman from West Covina, that he might have eaten something bad at lunch. He was giggling by the time he got home. Learning about computers was for schmucks and losers. He had the gift of sales genius. He didn't need to learn programming like some fool at a credit bureau.

Lenny and Linda went about their lives in a fashion which did indeed superficially resemble the way they had lived before 'ludes. The big difference was that Lenny and Linda felt a lot of anxiety a few times each day. Usually they would come in the morning or after lunch or maybe during a lull in dinner-table conversation. "They" were small darts of worry or fear or even stark terror. When "they" came around, Lenny and Linda would exchange looks if they were together. If they were alone, they would not look at anyone. Then they would dive into pocket or purse and dig out a 'lude. Just holding the large white pill in their hands made them feel better. They would touch it for a few minutes, and then they would swallow it. Lenny and Linda both learned pretty quickly how to swallow a 'lude without water. Sometimes, if Lenny or Linda were really eager to go into hyperspace and leave old man terror behind, Lenny or Linda would break the 'lude in half or even into quarters. They had learned quickly that the absence of pain arrived just a little sooner when the pill was broken up.

Then Lenny and Linda would go back to doing just exactly what they were doing before they took the pill. Their faces might be numb and their speech would be slurred, but in most circles in Los Angeles, that would hardly be noticed. So Lenny and Linda went on about their lives as if they were the same people. But, in fact, they now operated almost completely Quaalude by Quaalude, and without much else to get them through the day.

Within a month, they were so completely captured by fear about what would happen to them without the 'ludes, guilt about being at the very least "habituated" to a drug, and terror of what the future held for them without money or self-respect, that they were shadows of their former selves. Linda, who might have been expected to resist the allure of the drug, liked it every bit as much as Lenny did. By taking it, she could take away the image in her mind of Lenny on the cross and herself weeping beneath it. That was worth something. Lenny would have flown into little pieces without the drug—or so he believed—and so it became more a matter of need than of liking for him.

But as I said, Lenny and Linda did superficially resemble other middle-class young couples. After all, a man with an artificial heart looks to the outside world just like any other man. By the exact same token, Lenny and Linda seemed to be like other L.A. couples. The drug is so subtle and clever that it allows its users to function roughly normally while still craving the tablets more and more frequently. Unlike what you might imagine, the Quaalude addict does not lie around in alleys in Harlem waiting for a fix. He goes about life like most people, with the main exception that he does not consider anything as important as getting that 'lude. Once he has it, he can talk, do long division, drive a car, shop at a store, all more or less. Of course, he has lost a crucial edge which successful people generally need, but most people did not have that edge, anyway. Lenny did, but he lost it the night he first started taking 'ludes. Without it, he was much like most people.

Except, except, except. Except that he would have committed murder to get more Quaaludes. Except that he was completely off the track of achievement and on the track of self-destruction. Except that his life had turned from paradise into hell.

Naturally, Lenny had lost the ten-thousand-dollar deposit he had given the Hungarian. The man had toyed with the fringes of a prayer shawl while he sneered at Lenny. "This is not a business for little children or for fools," he said. "You made a bargain with me. Part of the bargain is that the deposit is mine. I gave you a very good price on the building. If you do not go through, the contract says I keep the deposit. That is law."

Joel was far more generous. He told Lenny that he sympathized and that it would take some doing, but somehow he would get somebody else to buy out Lenny. "It's possible that you might even come out ahead, because that disco is going to be a little money factory and people are dying to get in." In a few weeks, Lenny was indeed bought out and even came out five thousand dollars ahead. The money went instantly to pay off Master Charge. Lenny suffered humiliation worth a billion dollars for having to back out of the deal. Joel told Lenny that he could get everything back, that a hustler like him could be bigger than ever. "But you ought to lay off the 'ludes for a while." Lenny promised that he would. He took two as he backed out of Joel's driveway.

Lenny got rid of the airplane, returned some toys from a hi-fi store, and drastically cut back on his meals out. In fact, Lenny's financial situation was soon extremely poor, but no longer the material of suicide files. But since the real problem had always been in Lenny's mind and not on a balance sheet, the liquidation of assets and debts made Lenny feel worse instead of better. He had now "actualized" his failures by discarding, involuntarily, the tokens of success. He told people that he was simply "straightening out my life so I can have more time for the really important things," but he did not mean it. He had only one important thing in his life by this time, anyway.

Friends who knew Lenny and Linda and whom I knew often ask me how Lenny and Linda could have become so deeply involved with Quaaludes so fast. The answer is not complicated. How long does it take to pick up a fifty-dollar bill? How long does it take to grasp happiness out of anxiety? When you have seen Shangri-La, how long do you have to be there to not want to return to Hoboken? And then, when the self-respect goes, too, the process is complete. Again, for Linda it was also a way of communing with her husband, but for Lenny, it was salvation. Against a real world of men in loud suits offering two-bit jobs if Lenny would agree to be castrated, Lenny had only one refuge: Quaaludes. They worked and nothing else did. The old Lenny might have picked himself up and found another job. But there was no more "old Lenny." That person had been wrecked by quick success and sudden death and the forbidden knowledge of a better way through chemistry. Lenny on Quaaludes was still a smart man with many ideas for how to manipulate the world through tricks and schemes. But to really achieve in this world, one needs a certain spark of energy which will drive one to actually *do* all the deeds one imagines. The Quaaludes rapidly smothered that spark, leaving only the clever plans and deals.

The Quaaludes also tended to erode the quality of Lenny's judgment about the most basic and crucial areas of his life. For example, while he actually rationalized his life in certain ways for the first few months after he became addicted to Quaaludes, lowering his indebtedness, living more frugally, abandoning his hopes of greatness overnight, he gradually began a course of action which eventually led to the severance of most of his remaining ties with respectability and certainly dashed any realistic hopes for a major comeback in the real-estate tax-shelter business.

Around November, Lenny began to feel that he owed a nice meal to Joel and Rochelle. He took them and Linda and me and my wife to La Scala. He tipped Tony fifty dollars and got the best table. He ordered three bottles of Taittinger La Francaise. He insisted that we all have after-dinner drinks. Then as a surprise, he told us that he was going to fly us all to Vegas to see Steve Martin's midnight show at the Sahara. Linda's mouth dropped open with shock. But Joel covered Lenny's bet immediately.

"Hey," he said, "I knew we couldn't keep this boy down for long. I knew that this boy was hot."

Lenny, drugged as he was, blushed and smiled like a schoolboy who has won a spelling bee.

"What's the deal?" Joel asked. "Is the shelter business back, bigger than ever? No, that's not it. You're into something new, something the rest of us haven't even begun to figure out yet. Right?"

"It's very hush-hush," Lenny said. "It involves plays in Eurodollars against oil-tanker shipments."

"I'm hip," Joel said. "All I ask is that you explain it to me sometime soon."

Lenny winked.

After the trip to Las Vegas, Lenny told me that it was all a joke, that he had read an article in the *Wall Street Journal* about plays on oil-tanker shipments and that was what put the idea in his head. "I like to give the impression that I'm in motion," Lenny said. "Even if nobody understands what you're doing, you want to make people think you're doing something, preferably something mysterious involving big bucks."

It all sounded like advice from one of Michael Korda's books, but if it helped Lenny, kudos to Michael Korda. Of course, it didn't help him at all. It did not confuse Joel or anyone else. In fact, it only confused Lenny, and confusion was the last thing Lenny needed at that moment. He was already so confused that he had written checks on the Century West Maintenance account for the entire evening at La Scala and at the Sahara, about six thousand dollars. He was so further confused that he also wrote a check on the same account to buy Linda a diamond and gold bracelet at Tiffany's in Beverly Hills and the selfsame account to pay off his American Express bill in full. By the time he was even with American Express, he was into the Century West Maintenance account for about twenty thousand dollars.

"That's nothing," Lenny said. "When the business opens up again, we'll be doing a helluva lot more business than that every day. I don't think Max is going to hold it against his best salesman and his partner that I borrowed a little money for a few months. Max thinks bigger than that. Anyway, I put my check for the whole amount in our safe-deposit box at the bank just to show Max I mean to keep everything even."

That's what I mean about bad judgment. Lenny would never have thought that a check stuck away in a safe-deposit box meant a thing before he started with 'ludes. Now, he had convinced himself that he had simply exchanged one form of money for another. In fact, he had exchanged something for nothing. The people who give up the something usually do not like the people who give up nothing, as Lenny was to learn. Not only that, but Lenny would never in his alert days have imagined that he could embezzle money and not get caught.

"Listen," he said, "this girl at the office who keeps the books really likes me. She's always asking me to come over and help her put up pictures at her apartment and that stuff. So maybe she'll catch it, and then if she does, she'll tell me first and I'll get it hushed up. She really likes me."

Lenny told me that one day while we ate cheeseburgers at Carney's, a converted railroad car which sells cheeseburgers smothered in chili right on Sunset Strip. Next to us, an angelic little girl with blond hair and red lips smiled at us over french fries. She wore a

T-shirt that said "Life Sucks." I told Lenny that he had better tell Max about the whole thing right away and offer to pay him back little by little.

"No possible way, man," Lenny said. "That's not my style at all. Max knows I'm the best salesman he's ever had. He's not going to go apeshit over a little thing like this."

Naturally, it turned out later that the same girl who kept the Century West books was also Max's mistress, and that she felt her first loyalty to the man who had bought her a condo at Venice Beach, not to mention a Porsche Turbo Carrera, and not to a good-looking guy who worked for her keeper.

When the check came into the office one day made out to Tiffany for $6,852, signed by Lenny Brown on the account used to buy Pine-Sol, Marlys, the little bookkeeper of Century West, took it right to Lenny. At that moment, Lenny was reading an article about the menace of sleeping-pill abuse. (I have noticed that drug addicts are always fascinated by any literature on their particular drug. I have also noticed that drug addicts are very often health-food nuts. It all hangs together perfectly, since both interests are signs of complete absorption in self, as is drug addiction in the first place. This is not to say that many drug addicts are not fine people who are interested in others occasionally. But the compulsion to drug oneself is clearly a sign of overwhelming interest in self. Reading about oneself and taking exotic foods for oneself are also signs of narcissism, but on that, more later, I am sorry to say.) The little bookkeeper Marlys strolled over to Lenny, blew a cloud of Pall Mall smoke in his face, and laid the check down gently in front of him. "Are you playing some kind of joke, Lenny?" she asked.

Lenny stared at the check and said, "Let's just keep this to ourselves, OK? I needed to buy something and I didn't have my regular checkbook. Maybe we can get this straightened out and not tell anyone, OK?"

Marlys had worked as a real-estate saleswoman in south Philadelphia before she got the good thing going with Max Sherman. She was not particularly beautiful, and she had an irritable personality. She knew only that she was completely set with Max Sherman and that she did not want to rock the boat. Still, she had those light blue eyes which sometimes indicate insanity, so she was willing to take a small chance on Lenny. "Listen," she said in a low voice, "you go home and get your checkbook and write us a check for this before the bank closes today, and we'll be golden. Otherwise, I've got to tell Max." She raised her thick eyebrows in mock conspiracy and walked away, swiveling her hips. Lenny was not eager to take up that particular offer. He simply loved Linda too much to be seriously interested in anyone else.

But Lenny did realize that he might be in a spot. As I said, this was another occasion when his judgment was impaired by the drug. A year earlier, he would have laughed at this idea, and yet he did it. He went home, got his checkbook, and gave a check to Marlys for the amount of the bracelet. "Here we go," he said. "Even steven."

"I hope you're not jerking me around," Marlys said, playing with her ponytail. "I could get in a lot of trouble if this bounces."

"I don't think this is going to bounce," Lenny said. He laughed a falsely confident deep-throated laugh, and then he went out to lunch.

The check could not have cleared if it had wings. Lenny's account was already overdrawn by at least a thousand dollars before Lenny wrote the make-believe check to Century West. The bank was no longer prone to honor Lenny's overdrafts for ten dollars, not to mention seven thousand dollars, more or less. Marlys was a smart girl in the bookkeeping department. She called the bank as soon as Lenny left for lunch. While Lenny ate veal paillard at the boutique of La Scala, Marlys learned from Marcia, the assistant cashier at the Commercial Bank of California, that Lenny's account could not bear a check for ten cents, let alone Lenny's make-believe heavyweight check.

What on earth could have made Lenny do such a thing? Adam Smith could not explain such self-destructive behavior, but I suspect that Sigmund Freud could. The drug had made Lenny feel so bad about himself (except, of course, while he was high) that Lenny wanted to actually harm such a bad person. The check episode was simply a way of validating his own judgment of himself. That was a possibility.

It was also possible that Lenny was so deluded from the drug and from his relentless escapes from reality that he could no longer clearly tell what he was doing. At some point (Linda once told me),

Lenny began to behave as if he were a spectator in his own life, as if
he were simply watching a movie of his rise and fall. I have known
people who were so pained by the truth of their lives that they could
only get through each day by pretending that they were no more
than observers of their lives. I am told that terminal cancer patients
sometimes develop this attitude. Lenny might well have wanted the
amusement value of seeing a self-destructive fool—played by someone he knew well—actually take his career and tear it into small
pieces right in front of his eyes. He might have thought that catastrophe would befall the stage Lenny, the Lenny on-screen, but that he,
the spectator Lenny, would simply have a good laugh.

At any rate, Lenny's check did not clear. Lenny had two 'ludes
with Joel at lunch and did not feel anything except that he wanted to
go home and play with the dog, Daisy. He did not even think about
the check. At some point that afternoon, Marlys reluctantly told
Max about the check, and about a few others she had discovered
while she was at it. There was one for renting an airplane, a few for
meals at La Scala, and even several for repairs of a Mercedes convertible, not to mention a large one for accommodations and meals
at the Sahara. The total was about twenty thousand dollars. Max told
Marlys to tell no one about the whole episode. It could seriously
erode investor confidence in the entire Century West structure.
Then he asked Marlys when he could take her to the small apartment he had rented for her at Lake Arrowhead. His wife was at a
marathon seminar in fund-raising techniques for the Women's
League for Israel, and he would be free for the whole weekend.

After Marlys left the room, Max started to pace up and down. He
was hysterical with anger. When he thought of the betrayal of trust,
he could scarcely control himself. Still, he had to watch his blood
pressure, and still he would surely get even with this young sonofabitch. That would make his systolic pressure lower and get out a lot
of anger. The doctor had told Max not to hold it in. Max would blow
Lenny right out the fucking window. How dare the little prick, after
Max had practically taken him out of the gutter and treated him like
a son? The total putz had been wearing shiny pants when Max met
him. Now the little asshole was getting better tables than he did at
fancy restaurants. Yes, indeed, the boy was due for some very strong
lessons. Plus, the kid was on something. That was for sure. He

wasn't even at work most days. The other days, he was totally wasted. He could hardly focus his eyes. He giggled when Max saw him across the room at Le Restaurant. Yes, sirree, that boy was in for some major lessons in whom not to make a fool of.

While Max was engrossed in thoughts of revenge, Lenny sat by Joel's swimming pool and spun a wholly fanciful tale of his adventures speculating in interest rates on Eurodollars. Without question, he assured Joel, this kind of transaction, handled in total secrecy by brokers in Zurich, would make Lenny a force to be reckoned with in finance.

Joel had recognized that Lenny was pulling his chain for a good long time now. But Joel had long ago put Lenny into the category of people whose main value is amusement. Lenny could tell all the tales on earth about margin speculation in ten million Swiss francs at a time, and Joel would simply smile and feel lucky that he knew better. Joel also liked to give Lenny 'ludes, although not all the time, because Joel liked to see Lenny when he was fucked up. Lenny was even funnier when fucked up than when straight. And if Joel could get Lenny and Linda fucked up, they would start making out in front of him. It was almost like having a live sex act, all for the price of a few 'ludes. Plus, Joel felt as if he were the lord of a castle, and he had these two kids to be his fools. Really, Lenny was pretty amusing when he was out of his mind on 'ludes.

None of this means that Joel was a fiend. He had real feelings for Lenny. He often offered to lend him money. Many times, he offered to help Lenny get a new job. Lenny always turned him down. Joel offered to take Lenny and Linda to Ma Maison or La Scala anytime he went. Joel would have liked for Lenny to succeed at Century West Equities. But if Lenny was going to fuck up his life for good, Joel felt he had paid for a choice seat. If you think that this shows a cruel streak in Joel, I would ask you to find twenty people without that streak, five in L.A.

After a few hours, Joel had to leave to visit one of his car washes. Lenny was too far gone to walk. He struggled over to the pool house. He sat in a wicker chair and turned on the TV. It played a syndicated rerun of Bob Newhart. Lenny watched for a minute and then fell asleep. Who knows what dreams doomed men dream? It was enough for Lenny that he was asleep.

He awoke because Rochelle had come into the room. She had

taken off her black maillot and loosened the band around her hair. She had also begun to kiss Lenny's neck. Rochelle had always liked Lenny. Although most would not have called her the motherly type, nevertheless, she was fond of thinking of Lenny as her little boy. He needed her help. While Bob Newhart talked to a dentist next door, Rochelle ran her smooth, beautiful hands across Lenny's chest. He started to shift in his chair. When she ran her hand across the lap of his trousers, Lenny awakened.

"Jesus," he said. "What're you doing?"

"Don't talk," Rochelle said. "Talking doesn't help. Kisses, Lenny." She began to kiss him. He kissed her, too. Then he shook himself like a dog after a bath.

"I can't, Rochelle," he said. "It isn't right. We're all friends."

Rochelle lowered herself into Lenny's lap so that her breasts were flush with his face. "Forget it, Lenny," she said. "This is just between us. It has nothing to do with anyone else."

"I'm sorry, Rochelle," Lenny said. "But it just can't happen. I'm sorry."

She started to kiss him again, and then he gently, firmly pushed her away. She stood up. He stood up. "I've got to go now," he said. She crooked her arm and her leg and smiled at him. He kissed her on the cheek.

"I can't believe you, Lenny," she said. "There's no way you should even be in this town. You just don't get it at all."

"I'm sorry," he said.

"Don't be sorry," she said. "That's why I like you. If you were another manipulating scumbag like Joel, I wouldn't touch you." She hung her head in sorrow, and then she said, "I'll break up with Joel, soon. It's just that it's hard out there by yourself."

She said that, and then she walked out of the room and dove into the pool. Lenny watched her for a moment and then walked out, through the house, out onto the sprinklered lawn, and into his car. He started it and drove away. His head was spinning with confusion. The check which would sink his career was completely absent from his thoughts. He hoped that he had done the right thing about Rochelle. She surely looked wonderful, with those gourdlike breasts and those tiny features. But if there was one polar star in Lenny's life, one thing that allowed him to get out of bed in the morning, it was his complete loyalty to Linda. Nothing was worth losing that feeling of pride that he still did one thing right. Still, she had looked good.

Maybe it would be good to be in a slightly structured environment after all that craziness, Lenny thought. So he headed through the traffic on Whittier Drive to Century City. He was a murderer return- ing to the victim's body while the police were still on the scene. In his drama, however, he was both murderer and victim.

Max had locked Lenny's door and put a note on it saying, in typescript, "See me." Lenny was so blitzed, so willfully eager to end his career in Los Angeles, that he thought perhaps Max was going to tell him that he would start selling tax shelters again tomorrow. After all, there had been rumors that the business was about to break wide open. He did not even think about the bounced check.

When Lenny strolled into Max's office and plopped himself down in the corner of Max's leather couch, Max could feel his blood pres- sure rise. He had the nerve to still act like everyone was buddy- buddy after all this shit? He had the crazy daring to do that?

"Don't sit down," Max said in a hissing growl. "You're not going to be here long enough to sit down." His voice was so harsh that Lenny snapped out of his reverie as if he had been given a shot of adrenaline right into his coronary artery. "In all my life," Max said, "I have never treated anyone the way I treated you. I have a son, a fine boy in his third year at Northwestern, and I don't treat him as well as I treated you, to my eternal shame. You were hungry and I fed you. You were poor and I made you rich, if you hadn't fucked everything up as I assume you have. You were just a fucking atom floating in space, a total nothing, a guy who was so far out to lunch you couldn't find McDonald's with a searchlight on Ventura Boule- vard. You were fucking drowning, man, and I offered you a life jacket."

Max was letting it all out, but he was not feeling any better. In fact, he felt worse. He paused for a moment to feel the pulse on his neck, the way Doctor Westin had told him to. His face was flushed.

"Didn't I do anything for you?" Lenny said. "Wasn't I your best salesman?"

Max gulped. "You were a good racehorse, Lenny. I can't take it away from you. But Jesus H. Christ, you were just nothing until I gave you the chance."

"Didn't I make money for you?" Lenny asked. Like a man on trial for his life, Lenny suddenly recaptured his old eloquence, his sharpness that had been lost for months now. "You were a great friend to me," Lenny said. "The best I ever had. Didn't I do some things for you, for Century West? Did I make you ashamed of me? What's all this about? I didn't change the fucking law."

"Lenny," Max said, much calmer now for unknown reasons, "you stole. You stole from me who treated you like a son."

Lenny stared at Max and then stood up. "What the hell are you talking about?" he asked. "I have never taken one penny from you."

"You idiot," Max said, recovering his anger. "You think I authorized you to write checks to La Scala or to Tiffany or to the Sahara or for your American Express bill? That's stealing, Lenny. Stealing from the man who treated you like his son."

"I paid you back for those checks," Lenny said. "I just didn't have my checkbook with me."

"Lenny, you're already a thief. You gonna be a liar, too? Your checks are no good. They bounce as high as this office. You knew they were no good. What kind of shit is this, paying back with checks that aren't worth a nickel?" Max was subsiding again. His anger was genuinely mixed with sorrow and disappointment. He had actually loved this man who had stolen from him and lied to him. To Max, Lenny had actually been a younger, more vital reincarnation of Max Sherman. To have this other self turn against him was intolerably infuriating and also sad.

Lenny, to tell the truth, had also been fond of Max. Max had taken him from Hamburger Helper to Palm steaks. He had not intended to lie to Max (he told me later). He had forgotten that the checks he had given to Marlys were bad. This may seem impossible to you, a reader, but to a man who was up to a minimum of five or six Quaaludes each day, it was not impossible at all. He could have forgotten how to walk. So there Lenny stood, in front of Max, busted cold as a liar and a thief who had betrayed the only man who had ever trusted him with something really big. Lenny tried to act serious and contrite. He set his jaw. He started to talk in a deep voice like Tom Brokaw. And then he cried. Right in front of Max, he stood there on the plush pile carpeting and wept. Tears came out of his eyes and fell onto the floor which cost two dollars a square foot.

What did Max do? Max walked over to Lenny, put his arms around him, and wept, too. This may seem strange, since Max had just a few hours before vowed to kill Lenny. And, of course, Max was a businessman from whom money had been stolen. If this story had been a movie or a novel, Max would have hired goons to kill Lenny. If this were a movie or a novel, Max would have humiliated Lenny, ripped him up one side and down the other. Max would have been so furious about the loss of his money that he would have forgotten every consideration of affection or human feeling. But since this was real life and Max was a real person, he was far more troubled by the loss of a friend and a man whom he had thought of as a son. The money could buy his wife dresses at Bullock's Wilshire, and now it was gone. There would be more money. But Lenny had been part of him, and now Lenny was gone forever. He might not be dead, but he was as lost to Max as if he were dead, since he had wounded Max so badly that Max could not possibly admit Lenny to his heart again. To a TV watcher, this much affection on the part of one businessman to another businessman is incomprehensible. But Max Sherman cried and hugged Lenny, who had stolen from him and lied to him.

Then Max pushed Lenny away and said, "Listen, I'm sorry. But you've got to go. You're through in this business. You were like a son to me, but you stole. So I'll give you a little money to see you through, but just do me a favor and don't look for another job in this business. And don't come around here, Lenny. You did real bad."

Lenny looked at Max through reddened, tear-filled eyes. Then he stuck out his hand. Max looked at it, shook his head, and turned his back. Lenny smiled wryly and walked out of the office. He passed Marlys in the hall. "Thanks a lot, Marlys," he said.

Marlys said, "That's business, Lenny. I'm really sorry, but I have to buy groceries, too."

Lenny took from his office only a leather picture frame in which there was a picture of Linda in her bridal gown. He left everything else, including his Texas Instruments TI-84 business calculator. He had a KLH stereo desk-model radio which he had bought in his first week of work. He gave it to Ivory, a very tall black messenger who had always had a kind word for him when business was at its worst.

"Thanks, Lenny," Ivory said. "You going into some big deal where they gonna give you your own stereo built into the desk? I always knew you'd go on to something bigger and better than this. I always did know it. Lissen, Lenny, take me, too, OK? I'm going to L.A. Community College, and I can do a lot of things with computers. I'm learning FORTRAN. Not right now, maybe, but someday, you take me along, OK?"

"Of course," Lenny said. "Someday I'll be working for you. You're the one with the brains. I've got the looks."

"Now, you know that ain't true," Ivory said.

Lenny clapped him on the back, said he would take him to the Palm someday real soon, and then Lenny left. It is a measure of Ivory's humanity that he knew two hours before from Marlys that Lenny was broke, drugged out, and about to be fired. Lenny should have spent more time with Ivory and less with Joel.

There is no justice in the world, but there is poetry, especially tragic poetry. At the same moment that Lenny was leaving his office in Century City, Florence, the half-oriental ballet teacher, had a talk with Linda.

The rest of the waiters and waitresses with stars in their eyes had left. The room still smelled of their sweat. The room was overwhelmingly warm and still. Even though it was cool and dark on Melrose Boulevard, inside the studio it was hot and the light was pitiless. Florence looked carefully at Linda. To Florence, it seemed as if she had taken in a young, eager girl less than two years before and now had a broken-down, middle-aged woman. Linda did not hear the commands. She did not follow the music. She did nothing right at all any longer. Once, Florence had believed that Linda would soon be on toe. Now it looked as if Linda would be lucky to stay out of the grave.

Linda's white Jaguar was covered with nicks and dents. Linda's hands had burns and cuts on them. Her eyes were perpetually glassy. Until just a few weeks ago, she could go through the motions of pliés and relevés, but now she was a laughingstock, a living, pitiful joke. Florence had to glare at the other students constantly to keep them from snickering out loud at the girl who had once been the envy of the class.

"Linda, I'd rather you didn't come to class anymore until you get yourself cleaned up. I just can't take having you disrupt the class anymore," Florence said.

Linda was not Lenny. She stared at the floor and said nothing.

"I'm very sorry," came out as a whisper that Florence did not even hear. She, like her husband, began to cry. Florence, like Max Sherman, took her in her arms and hugged her.

"What happened?" Florence asked. "What drug are you on?"

"Quaaludes," Linda said in another whisper.

"Jesus," Florence said. "That's what I thought. Do you know how bad those things are for you? Don't you see what they're doing to you?"

Linda nodded. "I need them," she said simply.

"No, you don't," Florence said. Then she grasped Linda by the shoulders and said, "Your husband is making you take 'em, right?"

Linda shook her head. "No one makes me take them," she said. "No one. I take them because they make me feel a lot better."

"Are you crazy?" Florence asked. "Don't you see the way you look? Can't you tell you're a wreck?"

Linda lifted her face and looked at Florence. "Oh, God," she said, and then she sat on the floor and sobbed for fifteen minutes, convulsively, with her shoulders working back and forth.

"I just want you to know that you don't have to be like this," Florence said when Linda finally left. "I've seen people who stopped. They were happier people."

That night, Linda and Lenny sat and talked for an hour about how everything had turned to darkness. Once they had come to a new city, in rapture from the light, overwhelmed by the billboards, the cars, the palm trees. Now they were zombies, prisoners of their own prisons. In the jacuzzi, over the sound of the bubbling water, they talked about how they had set out a trap for themselves and then had fallen into it. The trap was that they had to be just as rich as the people on Roxbury Drive or else they would promise to torture themselves for the rest of their lives. The bait was the promise of feeling self-worth. The food in the prison was the daily knowledge that you had failed and that you were receding farther from your goals every moment. It was bitter fare.

Lenny and Linda talked about whether this would have happened to them in New York. Linda said no, that they would never have felt so driven, so compelled to be rich in a city in which you could see people in rags on street corners on Park Avenue. In New York, it was clearer that life went on even if you were not rich. But in Los

Angeles, where the only value at all was money, where no worth attached to any other activity except making money and displaying money, there would naturally be terror in not having a great deal of money. The very grass and asphalt of the city spoke of money and how only schmucks do not have it.

Out of this whirlpool had come the thoughts about what counts which now tortured Lenny and by osmosis tortured Linda as well. Not only had Lenny failed to make a lot of money. Not only was he surrounded by people who had made a lot of money. But also, he had become so addicted to a drug that he could not even think clearly anymore—except to know that taking the drug made it still more impossible to reach the house on Roxbury Drive. And to make everything tidy, he had to take the drug to keep himself from feeling unbearable pain at having failed to have a tax-sheltered income of two hundred thousand a year.

After Lenny and Linda discussed how they had totally wrecked their lives by falling into a trap made for themselves by themselves, how their values were totally and completely fucked up, how they would be better off dead than living the kind of life filled with terror and self-hate that they now lived, they took showers, dressed, went into North Hollywood to have a pizza, and then went over to a certain Robert's house and bought fifty Quaaludes. The pain of knowing just how badly they had ruined everything made them need a drug to blot out the knowledge, just as a suicide often kills himself in contemplation of death.

Still, that night something was born in their minds. That night was the first time Linda had ever fully realized how badly off they were and how urgently she needed to get out of the pit. Lenny, for the first time, realized that if he did not make a drastic change, there was no future at all. After the incident with Max, after seeing and hearing how unhappy Linda was, he could not even pretend that things would get better unless he did something drastic. The road they were on led to skid row, literally, or else to an early death. There had to be some kind of major change.

LOS ANGELES,
SUMMER, FALL, AND WINTER 1978-1979

PILGRIMAGES

You may have wondered how Lenny Brown got his Quaaludes. After all, you cannot simply go to an Alpha-Beta and buy Quaaludes. You have to get them through painful, strange channels. Even the wealthiest, most resourceful studio head has problems keeping himself well supplied. For a man who is in constant fear about money, who is confused and depressed even without the Quaaludes, who suffers from shame and mortification on a continuing basis throughout the day except when he is under the influence, who needs the drug desperately to keep a shark of self-hate from devouring him altogether, the quest for Quaaludes is torture.

Yet it was this growing torture, in addition to the disintegration of every other part of Lenny's life, which eventually led to Lenny and Linda's giving themselves a new lease on life. Like patrons of a movie theater watching a terrible movie, they eventually became so revolted by the movie which was their lives that they walked out of the theater. But a crucial part of that movie is just how Lenny kept himself and Linda supplied with 'ludes and just why January 16, 1979, in a shack in Venice, Lenny reached the breaking point.

This is how Lenny Brown got Quaaludes. At a certain point which I do not remember, it became too embarrassing for him to get them from Joel. There are negative value judgments attached to asking a friend for eight Quaaludes a day, although Joel was happy to oblige. Lenny had no idea of where to look first, but he knew that people in need of medication go to doctors. That was Lenny's first post-Joel route.

Dr. Herbert Wallerstein was listed in the Century City Neighborhood Phone Book as an internist and a medical corporation. His office was just a block from Lenny's. Lenny phoned one morning, told the woman who answered the phone that he "had been having some headaches and trouble sleeping lately," and got an appointment for that same afternoon. He was frightened, and so he asked me to come with him.

His appointment was for three-thirty. Lenny did not want to be late, so he left his own office a little after three. He stopped to get some gum at the newsstand downstairs. As he rummaged through his sports-coat pocket for change to pay for the gum, Lenny found a real treasure: half a 'lude. Left over from God knows when. Lenny crushed the pill in his mouth, chewed it, then covered up the familiar bad taste with a stick of sugarless cinnamon-flavored Trident. Fortified for his appointment, Lenny Brown hit the street. It was the first time he had walked anywhere for a long time. We passed a lot of pretty girls in tight jeans as we walked across the wide pedestrian bridge that spanned the Avenue of The Stars. Lenny spotted a drugstore in the lobby of a nearby office building. Perfect, he said. After he got his prescription from Wallerstein, he would just walk over there and get it filled. No problem.

Wallerstein's waiting room was packed. None of the people waiting looked sick. The half 'lude kicked in. I could see Lenny's eyes glaze over. He pulled himself together, lighted a Viceroy, a habit he had picked up as he entered the Land of Nod, and approached the receptionist.

"I'm Lenny Brown," he said. The woman did not bother to look up from her appointment book, thinly ruled pages in an elegant leather binder. That, and a Rolodex, were the only items on the blond oak parson's table that served as her desk.

"You're smoking," said the receptionist. The tone in her voice made Lenny look around for an ashtray. There was none to be found. The receptionist looked up from her book with a big phony smile. She handed Lenny an ashtray which was actually from a McDonald's restaurant, made of shiny, red tin, with an embossed M in the middle. "Use this," she said grimly. "If you must."

"Yeah," said Lenny. "I've been meaning to quit." He stubbed the just lit butt out in the shabby disposable receptacle and voluntarily placed the mess on the edge of the parson's table.

"You're three-thirty," the woman said. She was in her late forties, her hair already gray, pulled in a tight bun. There was a pencil in her hair. "I'm afraid we're a little backed up."

"I hope it's not going to be too long." Lenny made a big show of looking at his watch. "I've gotta be back at the office . . . well, as soon as possible." The receptionist had dealt with people in a hurry before, people who looked at their watches exactly like Lenny Brown. She actually looked as if she enjoyed it.

"There doesn't seem to be a seat for you, Mr. Brown," she said. "Let me see if I can rustle one up."

The receptionist brought Lenny a fold-up director's chair which she placed right next to her own desk, as if he had been bad in class and had to sit next to the teacher. I sat on a couch arm. As soon as a regular seat opened up, he took it. Lenny sat on a long white wicker couch between two middle-aged women with identical black shopping bags from Maxfield Bleu.

A little boy sat in the matching wicker armchair to Lenny's left, wearing a brightly striped rugby shirt and painter's pants. He apparently belonged to the woman seated directly to Lenny's left.

"Jason," the woman said. "Stop fidgeting. Read a magazine or something."

"But Mom," the kid whined, "we've been here for three hours."

"Three hours ago," the mother pointed out, "you still had two hours left of school. I picked you up an hour ago. We've been here less than forty-five minutes."

The boy could not fight reason. He picked up the current issue of *Architectural Digest* and leafed through it. As he did, he crossed his legs, assuming the posture of a thirteen-year-old guest on the "Dick Cavett Show."

"Mom," he said after a while, holding the magazine open to a spread that Lenny could see was titled "The Total California Lifestyle." "Isn't this the house Dad was gonna buy?"

The woman examined the glossy color pages. "No," she said, after a cursory examination. "The house we were looking at had a tennis court."

"Right," said Jason and was quiet. The waiting room emptied a little. A couple of people were called and their business completed in short order.

It was three fifty-five. Lenny told me he was getting a headache. Staring at the Miró print on the opposite wall would not make him feel any better. Random color, random lines. The signature was the most interesting thing. The woman to his right, absorbed in the second third of a paperback edition of *The Godfather*, did not hear her name the first time it was called by the receptionist. "Mrs. Berkowitz," the receptionist repeated in gentler tones, "the doctor will see you now."

Mrs. Berkowitz marked her place in the novel by turning down a page corner and walked by the receptionist into the inner office. As she passed the parson's desk she said to the nurse, "Did you hear that Tara was accepted at Smith?" Lenny closed his eyes. He sighed and slid to his right along the couch for more room. "I'd better be next," he said.

He was. As Lenny approached the door he pressed the heel of his right hand against a throbbing temple and paused for a moment. He whispered, "Oh, God."

"You *do* look tired, Mr. Brown." Herb Wallerstein was in his early fifties. His hair was appropriately salted with gray through the temples. He looked to be in good shape. Wallerstein was a couple of inches taller than Lenny and was lean and hard.

The men shook hands. "Please," Wallerstein said, "have a seat." Lenny sat in a leather slingback chair that he fleetingly remembered had been pointed out to him by Linda in a catalog from the Museum of Modern Art. Wallerstein did not sit down behind his desk, which was a thick sheet of tempered glass resting on two huge slabs of Italian marble. Instead, he chose the Eames chair in the corner.

The doctor pulled at the knees of his gray flannel slacks, straightening the creases. He unbuttoned the middle button of his blue Brooks Brothers blazer, letting the jacket fall free, revealing a blue oxford-cloth Brooks Brothers shirt and an understated repp tie. Lenny became conscious of his own more casual attire: a dark-blue sports coat, double-vented, a collarless blue and white pinstriped sports shirt. Calvin Klein. The top three buttons undone. Things had changed since he had moved to Los Angeles.

Lenny told me about the conversation with the doctor.

"I'm told that you have been experiencing some head pain?" Wallerstein prodded. "Also insomnia?"

"That's right," said Lenny. "Sometimes, it's like, well, suddenly my whole *body* tenses up, like a coil or something."

"And when does this generally occur?"

"Well, I get these headaches sometimes in the late afternoon. I have one now, as a matter of fact. The tenseness happens at night. Sometimes I have a rough time sleeping."

"When was the last time you had a physical checkup, Mr. Brown?"

"In New York. My wife and I moved out here a while ago. The doctor said I was OK. In great shape, as a matter of fact."

"So," said Wallerstein. "These headaches and the sleeplessness, they are a Los Angeles phenomenon?"

"I guess so," Lenny said. He tried a small laugh. Lenny thought Wallerstein was making a joke.

Wallerstein did not smile. He stood up and shot his cuffs. "I think the best thing to do, Mr. Brown, would be for you to see Lucy here in my office and make an appointment for a complete physical. Then we can find out what's what."

"Actually," Lenny said carefully, "I don't think there's anything really wrong with me."

"Then why," asked Dr. Wallerstein, "come to me in the first place?"

"A friend of mine," Lenny said, "actually, a guy who works in my office, he was sort of having the same problem. Probably due to all the smog out here. Anyway, he had these pills that he took, just once in a while, but they really seemed to help. I forget what they were called. He gave me one once. Normally I wouldn't take pills from friends, but I had real bad headaches, that tense feeling, and the pill really cleared things up." Lenny talked like a little boy, out of nervousness and a desire to con the doctor.

"Yes," said Wallerstein. "And you can't remember the name of this pill? I must warn you, Mr. Brown, I am not a big believer in medication. Usually, doctors these days are treating only the symptom. I like to get at the root of the problem, so to speak."

"I think the pill started with a Q," Lenny mused. "All I really remember is that it was big, a big white pill. I remember that," Lenny confided, "because it was really hard to swallow. I'm not used to taking pills, I guess."

Wallerstein sighed for a full minute. "Could the name of the pill possibly have been methaqualone? Or maybe just Quaalude? Could that have been it, Mr. Brown?"

"Yeah," said Lenny. He pretended to think for a minute. "Yeah. I think that was it. In fact, I'm pretty sure."

"You want me to give you a prescription for, say, fifty Quaaludes, Mr. Brown?" the doctor asked. "Shall we see if the pills do the trick for you?"

"Well," said Lenny, his spirit soaring, "it might be worth a try. Then, if they don't work, I can come back for the physical. We could try something else."

The doctor turned to Lenny. "Mr. Brown," he said as he removed his glasses, "do you mind if I ask you a question?"

"Not at all," said Lenny.

"Do you think that you can come in here with your eyes spinning around in your head and tell me that someone gave you a pill and you can't remember the name, and I am going to give you both the name *and* the pills? Do you think that I would give you the pills without a complete physical? Do you think that I am insane? Your presumption is almost unbelievable. Unbelievable." Wallerstein was almost screaming.

"I don't understand," Lenny said. "What are you writing? I mean, I do have these headaches."

"Look," said Wallerstein. He appeared calmer now. He ripped off the bottom portion of a prescription slip, just the white paper part, not the part with his name and number on it. He kept the top part on the pad. "Go see this guy," Wallerstein said. "A colleague of mine." Wallerstein said the word "colleague" the way Hitler said the word "Jew." "You're going to get the pills somewhere, and it might as well be from him. He needs the business."

Lenny took the slip of paper. He was silent. Wallerstein had written the name of a Dr. James Dolan. He had a telephone number with a Silver Lake exchange, a long way from Century City.

"See Lucy on the way out," Wallerstein said. Lenny was almost out of the office. "Mr. Brown?"

"Yes?" Lenny turned.

"I'm sorry I raised my voice. I didn't mean to lose my temper. It's been a long day."

Why should he stop and see Lucy? Lenny wondered. He was not going to have a physical, at least not with Dr. Wallerstein. He walked past the adjacent office.

"Mr. Brown," a voice stopped him from inside.

"Yes?"

"Could you come in here for a minute?" A severe young blond girl, also with her hair in a bun, appeared in the doorway. Lenny complied. "Have a seat," she said sweetly. "I'm just making up your bill for your consultation with Dr. Wallerstein."

Lenny watched her write for a few moments, then took the bill from her. It was for $200.

"The bill," Lucy said. "It's payable right now. That's the way we do it for these kind of consultations."

That was when Lenny realized that getting Quaaludes was going to be hard work.

"Hello. You have reached the medical offices of Dr. James Dolan. No one is in right now. Please leave your name, a message, and the time you called at the beep tone. Someone will get back to you as soon as possible. If this is an emergency, call six-six-six-oh-two-oh-two. Thank you . . . beep."

Lenny left his name, Wallerstein's reference, and both his home and office numbers. Lenny considered calling the emergency number, but he decided that could wait. If Dolan didn't return his call by nine o'clock, Lenny would try the emergency number. If he had read Wallerstein's tone correctly, Lenny's emergency was exactly the kind of emergency Dolan was talking about on his answering-machine message.

At nine-thirty, Lenny dialed Joel's number. When Joel answered, Lenny hung up. Self-respect was important. At nine-thirty, to Lenny Brown, self-respect was just as important as Quaaludes.

At ten o'clock the phone rang. A man's voice asked for Lenny Brown. There was music in the background.

"This is he," Lenny said.

"Lenny, Jim Dolan. You called?"

"Yeah," said Lenny. "Herb Wallerstein suggested I give you a call. Set up an appointment."

There was silence on the other end of the line. Then, "Herb *Wallerstein* told you to call me? Well," said the doctor, "well, that's fine, Herb told you to call. Went to school together, Herb and I. Damn fine internist." Lenny heard a woman's voice in the background. A whining voice.

"You know where my office is, Lenny?" Dolan asked. Dolan gave him directions.

"Would you like me to come at any particular time?" Lenny asked. Lenny hoped Dolan was a real doctor.

"How does ten o'clock in the A.M. sound to you?"

Lenny thought it sounded fine. But before he could tell Dolan, Dolan had hung up. Lenny assumed the appointment was firm. At any rate, he was busy with Century West Maintenance work for the rest of the day, then dinner with Joel and Rochelle.

Aaron Street ran up a steep, short hill. There were, perhaps, eight houses on the left side. The entire right side of the street was occupied by a long, yellow, slanted stucco structure that was called "Bora-Bora Plastics." A lunch truck was parked in front.

In the middle of the block, on the left, was a three-story Victorian house with a double driveway. A Mercedes station wagon, the first one Lenny had ever seen, was parked in the driveway. The other houses on the block were decrepit boxes, peeling paint; discarded television antennae lay crumpled on the lawn. Silver Lake flamingos. It was a long way from Roxbury Drive.

Lenny parked behind the Mercedes wagon and walked up the set of stone stairs which led to a carefully manicured walkway. He was in the right place. Dolan had actually hung out a shingle. It looked as if it had been made by a child with an elementary-school wood-burning kit.

Lenny stepped up onto an old-fashioned porch, the kind of porch young kids used to make out on in those fifties movies set in the South. He pushed the button and heard chimes. Lenny looked up and noticed a television camera hanging from a sandblasted, natural-wood rafter. The red light was on.

A voice came over the intercom. A sleepy man's voice. "Yes?"

"It's Lenny Brown," said Lenny. "I've got a ten o'clock appointment with Dr. Dolan."

"So you have," said the voice. "Listen, when you hear the buzz, push the door as hard as you can. Sometimes it sticks. If it doesn't open, buzz me again."

"OK," said Lenny. From somewhere he remembered that if the red light was on you were supposed to look directly at the camera.

Lenny heard the buzz and pushed hard. He exploded into the house. That day the buzzer worked perfectly. A grizzled tower of a man in a monogrammed bathrobe kept Lenny from falling on his face.

"Sorry I'm not dressed yet," Dr. Dolan said. "You're my first appointment. Want a cup of coffee?"

"No, thanks," said Lenny. He noticed that everything in the room, the large room that the small foyer led to, was covered in velvet. Not just the couch, but the walls, too. "I'm kind of in a hurry," Lenny said. "I've gotta get back to the office."

"OK, Lenny," Dolan said. "Here's how it looks to me. You look like a sensible guy. You look like you're in good health."

"I am," Lenny said. "I can't remember the last time I was sick."

"And you need some Quaaludes." Dolan shifted his buttocks in his desk chair. Lenny got the feeling he had made this speech before. "Now, Lenny," Dolan continued, "I'm sure you understand that I can't go around prescribing Quaaludes to every idiot who wants to get high. I've gotta protect myself. That's why, sometime soon, I'll need a medical history on you. See, I've got you in my file now. If the BNDD ever comes down on me, I'll have something to tell them."

"I understand," Lenny said.

"On the other hand," Dolan said, "I can't let this get out of hand. I can give you fifty per month."

"That's fine," Lenny said. It was an effort not to laugh out loud with glee. Dolan wrote out a prescription. He handed it to Lenny and stood up.

Lenny made a move to leave. "Lenny," Dolan said. "There's one more thing. I don't want you to get this filled at your regular drug-store. I want you to go to the Thrifty on Vermont and ask for Ralph. You know, a lot of pharmacies don't even keep Quaaludes in stock."

"Right," said Lenny.

"The other thing," Dolan said as he showed Lenny to the door, "are these office visits. I cost a hundred dollars each time. If you don't have cash now, that's OK. You look like you've got some money in your checking account. But from now on, it's cash, OK?"

Fifty Quaaludes lasted Lenny and Linda six days with strict, agonizing conservation.

Lenny called Dolan exactly a week after his first consultation. "How are you, Lenny?" Dolan asked.

"I'm all right," Lenny said. The tone of his voice made him an obvious liar. I was in the room and heard him and saw his face.

"Lenny, what's wrong?" Dolan asked.

"Jim," Lenny said. "Listen, I wouldn't ordinarily trouble you with something like this. The thing is, we've had a robbery. Some assholes just broke the glass doors in back and stole everything."

"Jesus," Dolan said, mock concerned.

"They got the televisions, Linda's jewelry, everything."

"You're insured?"

"Oh, yeah," Lenny said, "but it's the hassle. Plus, that feeling. We feel as if our most private lives have been invaded." Lenny could no longer sell tax shelters, but he could still sell better than most Presidents.

"I know what you mean, Lenny," Dolan said. "That's why I got the television. I hate having to do it, but I do."

"The weirdest thing, Jim," Lenny said, "is that they took the Quaaludes. They took all the pills. Linda had some Tetracycline for a cold, and they took that, too."

"You need another prescription, Lenny," Dolan said tonelessly.

"If it's possible, Jim. I know what you told me. But with the burglary, dealing with the insurance people . . . I don't know. I know I'll never be able to sleep."

"Where do you live, Lenny? Hollywood Boulevard? Above the Strip?"

"What a great memory you have," Lenny said, still selling.

"Well," said Dolan. "I'm going to be in the neighborhood around six o'clock this evening. I'll drop off a prescription. For a hundred this time. Maybe you should lock them up somewhere. Everybody's trying to get Quaaludes these days."

"Jim," Lenny said, "I don't know what to say. This is really terrific of you."

"No problem," said Dolan. "Hey, Lenny, do you know what time it is?"

"It's about two-thirty," Lenny said.

"Great," Dolan said cheerfully. "You've got time to go to the bank. It's gonna cost you two hundred bucks this time."

The visits to Dr. Dolan became more and more expensive as the fifty-pills-a-month limit disappeared. Within three weeks Lenny was paying two hundred dollars for each trip to Silver Lake and more for Dolan's trips to Hollywood, when the doctor was able to drop off the prescription. Getting the prescriptions filled was difficult, too. Lenny had to go to a certain pharmacist, a man named Ralph who operated out of a Thrifty Mart on Vermont Boulevard, not far from Dolan's office. Quaaludes were in big demand, motivated robberies, and not every drugstore stocked them.

Dolan had an arrangement with Ralph. I later learned that the doctor kicked back a few hundred dollars each month from his exorbitant fees for office visits, which made Ralph's risk worthwhile. Besides, Ralph only worked there. He did not own the place, so what the hell.

Sometimes Linda joined Lenny on his trips to Dolan or the Thrifty. She could tell how much he hated to go by himself. Especially at night. Lenny would always protest. "Linda," he would say, "you don't have to go. It's *twenty* minutes, a half hour at the most." Unfortunately, it was always longer. Sometimes the wait at the Thrifty would be almost unbearable, except that Lenny knew that if he just waited long enough he would go home with some Quaaludes. The people there, as opposed to the people in Wallerstein's waiting room, all looked very sick. Lenny hated for Linda to wait in the car outside of Dolan's house, but he was very glad for her company when he got out and it was time to head over to Vermont to get the prescription filled. At the Thrifty the couple roamed the discount aisles. Anything was better than sitting in white plastic chairs by the drug counter, next to poor sniffling old men in Salvation Army clothes, children with body-shaking coughs, junkies looking for a few Demerols to get them through the night. Lenny and Linda tried to look on the bright side of the Thrifty on Vermont. Sometimes, while they waited, they bought useless but cheerful things. Once, Linda bought Lenny a tiny rubber duck for the bathtub. Sometimes they would pick up a record album or two, or some cassette tapes. Recorded music was really cheap at the Thrifty. The best time to go was late at night because the store was not as crowded with poor people. Lenny and Linda both were depressed at the sight of Mexicans buying sneakers that cost $3.89 and were made to last less than a month. The customers at Thrifty looked as if the next stop was hell if they were lucky. Lenny, who was a sensitive guy, needed more 'ludes just to forget the Thrifty.

Around August, while brushfires burned all around Los Angeles, there was a crisis. Whenever Lenny called Dolan, he got nothing but the doctor's answering machine. He called around the clock, left more than ten messages in a two-day period. On the third day he got a different recording. The number had been disconnected. That night, Lenny and Linda went to the Thrifty to see Ralph. I had lunch with Linda a few days later, a late lunch on the Strip at the Old World, a place with rude service and bad food. Linda did not seem hungry that day. She looked tired. She looked as if she had not been out of the house for some time.

Linda told me that Ralph could not fill the prescription because Lenny did not have a current one. Also, the law had changed. Lenny needed a triplicate blank. Lenny had gotten to know Ralph fairly well, through many visits. Ralph had been a professional football player at one time. He had been on the third string of a team whose name Linda could not recall. "Anyway," Linda told me, "Ralph said that he hadn't heard from Dolan either, but he'd heard through the grapevine that Dolan had left town. It didn't surprise him. Ralph had been getting some phone calls about prescriptions for patients who didn't exist. Lenny thinks that Dolan was selling pills on the side, too."

Because Ralph liked Lenny, Ralph gave Lenny a phone number. The number belonged to Robert, an out-and-out Quaalude dealer in Hollywood. Lenny worried about going that far outside the law. The two had stood together in the parking lot of the Thrifty. Linda was in the car. Ralph wrote the phone number on the back of a movie-theater ticket. "Just tell him Ralph gave you the number and that you're cool."

"OK," said Lenny. He was nervous.

"Look," said Ralph, "you don't have to call him if you don't want to. I'm just trying to help you out here."

"I know," said Lenny. He got in the car with Linda and drove home. Then he called Robert.

A harsh male voice answered the phone. "Yeah?" said the voice. "What do you want?"

"Is this Robert?"

"Yeah, man, hurry it up. Who are you?"

Lenny introduced himself. He lied and said his name was Kenny. Kenny, a friend of Ralph's from the Thrifty. He said that he was cool.

"So what do you want, man?" Robert said. "Come on. I got things to do. You want coke? You want 'ludes? I got the best of everything. I'm sure Ralph told you that."

" 'Ludes," said Lenny. "I want Quaaludes." Robert's directness, especially on the telephone, made Lenny nervous.

"I don't have 'em," Robert said. Robert made a short barking sound, a strange laugh.

Lenny felt as if he had fallen into a hole in the earth and was being showered with thick clumps of dirt. "What do you mean?" was the only thing he could manage to say.

"Don't sound so sad," Robert said. "What I mean is I don't have them on the premises. I don't keep them here. I don't keep anything here. If the police come in, they'll find exactly nothing. How many do you want? What time can you be here?"

Lenny said, "I'd like fifty."

"*Fifty!* Come on, man!" Robert yelled. "Don't waste my time. A hundred's as small as I go."

"OK, then. A hundred."

"It'll cost you three hundred bucks. Cash." Robert gave Lenny his address, a big apartment building near Franklin and La Brea. "I have the penthouse," Robert said. "Apartment three-oh-four. It's on the third floor. Press the buzzer downstairs twice, two short buzzes, and I'll let you in."

"When do you want to do this?" Lenny asked.

"It's up to you," Robert said. "I'll be home for another fifteen minutes. Then I'm going out. I'll be back again in ninety minutes."

Lenny said, "I'll leave right now."

"All right. But if you're not here in fifteen minutes I'm leaving, anyway. I'm not going to wait around to turn a hundred Quaaludes. I've got things to do."

"Hey," said Lenny, on edge, "I said I'm leaving now. You can't live more than ten minutes from where I am."

Robert's building was easy to find. It was a three-story crackerbox with underground parking. Lenny got buzzed in right away and waited in a trash-filled lobby for the smallest, dirtiest elevator he had ever seen. Lenny guessed the building was populated mainly by hookers. There were mirrors everywhere he looked, the distinctive mirrors with fake marbling in them.

Robert's apartment door was partially open. Lenny knocked, anyway. "Come on in," Robert said, appearing in the doorway. He was in his early twenties, skinny, and never looked anyone (at least not Lenny) directly in the eye. "I told you I was in a hurry."

It was a small apartment. A pigsty. Empty lemonade containers and *Hustler* magazines were scattered all over the peeling linoleum floor in the tiny kitchen. The only uncluttered spot in the room was the kitchen counter. There was a professional Rohm and Haas triple-beam scale for weighing cocaine and ten rows of Quaaludes, ten in each row, in neat straight lines.

"You got the cash, man?" Robert said. "Come on, let's see it." Lenny removed three one-hundred-dollar bills from his billfold (cash obtained from a loan at twenty-two percent from a loan company which advertised in the *Los Angeles Times* classified section). Robert promptly snatched the money from his hand. "You want these in a bag?" Robert asked. He referred to the 'ludes.

"Sure," said Lenny.

Robert opened a kitchen drawer. Lenny could see the drawer was stuffed with plastic baggies. Robert took one and scraped the Quaaludes from the counter. He handed the bag to Lenny.

"Nice doing business with you, Kenny," Robert said. "You'll like these. They're the real thing. If you know anyone who wants to purchase a large amount, you can let me know. I'll cut you in."

At this time in Lenny Brown's life he thought that one hundred Quaaludes was a large amount. Robert almost pushed him out the door.

The first one hundred Quaaludes lasted Lenny and Linda nine

days with conservation that would have made Ansel Adams proud. Then Lenny tried to get in touch with Robert again. Robert's phone was busy for twenty hours. Once, Lenny tried an emergency break-through. The operator told Lenny that the phone was off the hook.

Finally, on the second day without 'ludes, Lenny reached Robert late at night. "You are a hard guy to get in touch with," Lenny said. He and Linda had canceled a dinner engagement that night so that they might be closer to a telephone, therefore closer to Robert. "Why don't you get an answering machine?" Lenny suggested.

"I don't need one," Robert said. "People can get in touch with me if they need to. Come on," he said, annoyed. "What is it? How many do you want?"

"Can you sell me a hundred and fifty?"

"What time is it?"

"It's eleven-thirty."

"Be here at . . . twelve-fourteen."

"Same price?"

"No," Robert said casually. "This is a new batch. They're boot-legs. But pretty good ones. I can't charge you as much for bootlegs as I can for real ones, can I? Let's see . . . I'll charge you two and a half a pill."

"Are these good?" Lenny asked.

"Look," said Robert, "I don't care if you want 'em or not. What the fuck is it gonna be?"

"I'll be there," said Lenny.

"If you don't like them," Robert said expansively, "you can bring them back."

Lenny hung up and got ready to go.

Dealing with Robert, Linda told me once, was always bizarre. First, there was Robert's craziness about time. ("Can you be here," he once asked Lenny, "in seven and a half minutes?") Second, there was the apartment itself, which was so filthy that Lenny never once allowed Linda to go up there with him. It was not like hanging out at the Thrifty, which was institutional filth. This, Linda told me, was personal filth. Lenny was always afraid of catching a disease. Like many drug addicts, he was obsessed with his health, either as a sign of narcissism or continued paranoia, if there is any difference.

On the other hand, Robert seemed to have his business in order.

He did not talk much, was always able to get pills within a half hour after Lenny reached him on the phone, and never delivered bad 'ludes. He even took the time once to explain very carefully to Lenny how to tell the difference between genuine 'ludes and bootlegs. And he was never himself seriously stoned. Robert took at most one or two pills a week. "There's no reason for us guys to take them," Robert said once. "What they're good for is for giving to chicks, right? Makes 'em wanna fuck, right? If we take 'em, it just makes it hard to get it up." Lenny always got out of Robert's as quickly as he could. He practically ran out of there that day.

Robert always seemed sure of himself. "If you're gonna deal," he said, "you've got to do it right. Always live in a security building, one with an underground garage. The garages always have a lot of good places to stash stuff, behind pipes, bricks, there's millions of places. Plus, you should never stay in one place for more than a few months. You've got to move around."

Lenny calculated that Robert had moved when his number was suddenly disconnected. He expected to hear from Robert at any moment with a new phone number, a new "penthouse" in a security building. Then he read in the paper about a dope bust in the Valley. There had been gunplay. A Robert Thornton, twenty-four, of Hollywood, was dead.

I am not exactly sure how Lenny got Quaaludes after Robert's death. Linda told me that one night soon after they had read about the bust, she and Lenny took a drive to the Thrifty on Vermont, to talk with Ralph. There was a new druggist behind the counter. He had never even heard of Ralph. "It's like he just vanished," Linda said. "Disappeared."

I suspect that Lenny made a new connection through someone he had met at Robert Thornton's apartment. I know that Lenny often met Robert at the Piece of Pizza restaurant on La Brea. I saw Lenny there once, after Robert's death. He was sitting with a large, red-bearded man in a camouflage jacket at an outdoor table. They were not eating pizza. A few nights later, shortly before the contretemps of the bad checks, Marlys, and Max Sherman, I was invited to dinner at Lenny and Linda's. The man with the red beard was there. Lenny and Linda were high. The man with the red beard did not stay for dinner. He left while Linda blended carrots for cream-of-carrot soup. She had become a gourmet cook, as if to offset her drug addiction with a meaningless (under the circumstances) accomplishment.

"It's really hard to keep this together," Lenny said, after his friend had left. "It's taking up too much of my time."

"What is?" I asked.

"Getting pills." Lenny looked dejected. "There's no one I can depend on. I've got to call at least six people every time I need some 'ludes. And a lot of times they're bad. Not just bootlegs, but bad bootlegs. Linda got really sick the other night, and I think it was from the new batch. It's getting so you can't trust anybody anymore."

"You should see all the numbers he's got crossed out in his phone book," Linda said. "It's ridiculous."

Now, just as Lenny's career at Century West was drawing to a close, forcing a change in his life, the chase for Quaaludes became excruciatingly painful. In a poetic way, the search for the drug would itself give Lenny a chance to be free of the drug. The confluence of forces was now moving against addiction and for hope. Occupational humiliation and drug-chase humiliation were building up irresistible pressure on Lenny and Linda.

An agitated Lenny Brown showed up at my apartment about a week after our dinner. Some time after the end of Century West Equities. It was almost midnight in January. "Come on," Lenny said. "Come on. I want you to take a drive with me."

Lenny did not look well. There were deep circles of black under his eyes, and his skin was very pale. "It's kind of late, Lenny," I said. "Why don't you come in for a minute? I'll make us some orange juice."

"No," said Lenny. "No, I've got to be someplace at twelve-thirty. It's right near here. Please," Lenny said. "Please come with me. I've got a lot of things to talk to you about."

"OK," I said. I was worried about Lenny.

"Listen," he said, as I locked my apartment door and we walked down the hall. "Would you mind driving? I've been driving all day."

"Not at all." We got into my car and drove.

"Head toward Hollywood," Lenny said.

"Lenny, where are we going?"

"A friend of mine," Lenny said. He gave me an address on Las

Palmas, near the Hollywood Bowl. When we got there, no one was home. Lenny pounded on the door of a small guest house. He could hear music inside. Still, no one answered the door.

"What time is it?" he asked me when he returned to the car.

"It's twelve thirty-five."

"Goddammit!" Lenny swore. "He said he'd be back by now. Would you mind waiting a few minutes?" Lenny got in the car. He sighed.

"I thought you wanted to talk," I said after a few quiet minutes had passed.

Lenny said up straight in his seat. "I've got a great idea," he said. "It's almost one o'clock, and this guy isn't home yet. Let's take a drive. We can talk while we're moving."

"Where do you want to go?"

"Venice. I know a guy in Venice. I think that's where the guy who lives here probably is."

"It's kind of late," I said. "Are you sure you want to do this?"

"Come on," Lenny said. "It's not *that* late, and besides, the freeway's gonna be empty this time of night. We're talking about a half hour, maybe forty minutes tops."

I headed down La Brea to catch the Santa Monica Freeway going west. We had gone only a few blocks when Lenny suddenly yelled, "Stop! Wait a second. Make a right here."

Lenny instructed me to stop outside of a Spanish-style multiunit stucco apartment building called the Hamilton Arms. I waited in the car. He was inside the building for more than fifteen minutes.

"What happened?" I asked when he got back in the car.

"Nothing." He seemed really disgusted now. "The guy let me have one Quaalude for ten dollars. He said that's all he had, but I don't believe him. He was jerking me off. I know he never has less than a hundred. But he's a real addict, and I guess he doesn't want to give up any personal stash."

"Are we still going to Venice?" I asked.

"I'm sorry I took so long in there," Lenny said. "Yeah, sure, let's go. If you don't mind."

We were cruising along the Santa Monica Freeway. Lenny had yet even to hint about what it was he wanted to talk to me about. He just sat there.

"Does Linda know where you are?" I wondered.

"Of course," Lenny said. "Well, I mean she knows I went out. She fell asleep really early tonight. Anyway, I think she might have been awake when I left. I'm not sure. Anyway, I left her a note."

Lenny's Venice routine was the same as his Hollywood routine. We went from house to house, knocking on doors. We woke up some people (Lenny was not sure of a couple of addresses), and some people were expecting Lenny. He got a couple of 'ludes here and a couple there. At two-thirty I was waiting in the car outside of a shack on the Venice canals. I had been alone in the car for thirty minutes. I could see shadows moving in the living room of the house where he had entered.

The front door of the shack opened wide. A man was standing in the doorway. "Come on in," he yelled to me. "Why don't you come in here for a minute?"

I pulled the Mercedes into the small sandy driveway and parked directly behind a rust-covered Sunbeam sportscar. The Sunbeam had no tires and sat unevenly on some homemade blocks. A For Sale sign was Scotch-taped to the trunk. No price was mentioned, just a phone number.

I got out of the car, locked it, and looked at my watch. It was two thirty-four. The only light on Liddie Canal, the small canal-front side street, came from an old-fashioned street lamp at the corner, thirty yards away. I looked up and saw ancient graffiti splashed in random and surprisingly bright colors on the rickety wooden fence that separated two shacks. There were peace signs, slogans, and posters of a smiling Gene McCarthy. He was running for President. The posters looked as if they had been put up yesterday, although I knew they had to be more than ten years old. I walked over to the fence and touched the corner of one McCarthy poster. It was stiff, fresh cardboard.

I heard the crunch of boots on gravel and turned around to see the shadow of a man walking toward me from the front porch of the house where Lenny had gone to buy Quaaludes.

"You're Lenny's friend," he said. The man was tall and fat. He wore light blue mechanic's overalls. He had long, curly blond hair. The grease on his forehead shone in the moonlight. He stood ten feet from me, next to a telephone pole which was plastered with posters announcing a rally sponsored by Another Mother for Peace. The rally was to be held in Griffith Park on a Sunday in April. April 1968. While I looked at the posters the man just stood there like a giant baby.

"I'm Daniel," he said finally. He made a motion with his hand that indicated I should follow him.

"Is there a problem?" I asked. We walked toward the house.

"The only problem is those fucking movie people hanging around here all the time," Daniel said over his shoulder.

"What do you mean?" I asked.

"They're shooting something here," Daniel muttered. "Something about the sixties, I guess. Are you blind or something, man? Didn't you see those McCarthy posters? Christ."

I had to step back when we walked through the open front door into the living room. The stench was overwhelming. A bare light bulb burned in the corner of the room. There were no people in there, only cats. Lots of cats. There were leavings of a dozen TV dinners scattered on the stained white carpet. A black cat with a white face abandoned a foil plate of dried-out macaroni and gnawed the laces of my shoes. Daniel kicked the cat against the wall.

"It's the only way to teach them," he said.

I heard voices from a back room. Lenny's voice and at least two others, perhaps three. I followed Daniel through an open doorway, and we were in a room which was completely dark. A couple of cigarettes burned in an ashtray on the floor by my feet. As my eyes adjusted to the darkness I could make out huddled shapes in the far corner. Some people were sitting around a mattress. One of them was Lenny. He was hugging his knees, rocking back and forth. He looked up and I thought he saw me, but he did not say a word.

"Lenny," I called out, wary of any movement in the darkness. I was trying for a conversational tone. "You about ready to go?"

Still, Lenny was silent. Daniel lit a match. We walked across piles of old newspaper. The walls were bare except for one poster, ripped from a magazine. It was a picture of cocaine in a Lalique crystal bowl.

"Something happened, man," Daniel said as we approached the group around the mattress. "Something bad happened."

Lenny stood. His hands were shaking. His eyes were dull and

looked right through me. I thought he was in shock. Then he tilted his head slightly, down toward the mattress. A young boy lay on his back. He was wearing cutoff jeans. I gasped. The top of his head was not there. It had been blown away. The bleeding had stopped. I guessed he had been dead for hours.

I took Lenny's hand and grasped it firmly. "Lenny," I said. I said his name over and over. The two men sitting on the floor did not look up. Finally, I got through. Lenny looked directly at me and made contact. Something had snapped in his eyes.

"Come on," he said. His voice was a whisper. "We've got to get out of here. These guys say they're going to call the cops. We should get out of here before the cops come."

A hand grabbed at my pants leg. A dirty, bearded face looked up at me. "We don't even know who he is, man," another shocked voice whispered. "We don't even know who he is."

Lenny said, "They say they found him tonight. They say someone just dumped him on the back porch."

The whisper at my feet got sharper. "Not *say*, Lenny. That's what happened. We just found him."

"That's right," Lenny told me. "They just found him."

"You remember that, Lenny," said the man at my feet. "We've never seen this cowboy before."

I held onto Lenny's hand. It was the only way to get him out of there. I led him through the living room and out the front door. I led him down the path, past the telephone pole, past the McCarthy posters. I had to physically put him in the car. By then, Lenny's whole body was shaking.

I drove down the one-way canal street out to Ocean, where I made a left and went up to Venice Boulevard. "Oh, God," Lenny moaned. I could hear the police sirens, then I saw the flashing red lights. There were three patrol cars. They did not seem to be in any great hurry.

"Oh, God," Lenny said. "Did you see that kid? Did you see that kid? He couldn't have been more than twenty years old."

I concentrated on the task of driving. I wanted to be home. I did not want to think about the spattered face of a young man. And I was worried about Lenny. He shook uncontrollably.

I drove down Venice to La Brea, then turned north toward Hollywood. When we were stopped for a light, Lenny reached into his pocket and fished out a plastic bag full of Quaaludes. He took out four of them and carefully placed them on his tongue. Then he chewed them dry. By the time we got to La Brea and Sunset, Lenny had stopped shaking.

LOS ANGELES
AND SANTA CRUZ,
WINTER AND SPRING 1978-1979
THE NEW AGE

Now flood that black gloom of Lenny and Linda Brown with shades of hopeful yellow and lines of promising, beckoning pink. The darkest hour is beginning to crack at the edges. Shafts of dazzling light, beaming down new beginnings and laughter, creep into focus to resurrect Lenny and Linda's life. Out of utter bleakness, out of the bottom of human misery, a sparkling sound of joy can just be heard, entering upon the stage of tragedy, upsetting all calculations of imminent doom.

When Lenny returned from that night in Venice, he sat in the front seat of the car muttering to himself that he was going to get out of this whole fucking, stinking business. "I'm not going to live like this," he said. "I don't care if Joel is rich and I'm poor. I don't give a single goddam about it. I'm getting out of it if I have to be a field hand."

We got home just as dawn was breaking off toward San Bernardino. He looked at me with bloodshot, frightened eyes and set his mouth in resolution. "I've been in a trance," he said. "Now, I'm getting out of the trance, and we're going to get moving on a few things so that Linda and I can get out of this pit."

Then he clapped me on the shoulder, a gesture from earlier, more confident days, and strode into the house, just as a poetic dawn appeared above the Petersen Publishing Company.

I later learned that he had surprised a fully awakened Linda, sitting in her nightgown, rocking slowly back and forth on the edge of the bed, moaning a low, soft moan like a prehistoric woman waiting for her man to come back from a dangerous hunt. "I was so scared," she told Lenny. "So scared. I thought maybe something like what happened with Robert had happened to you. I was really scared."

Lenny took her in his arms and soothed her the way you soothe a baby, bouncing her up and down, kissing the side of her neck. "It's all over," Lenny said. "We're through with that. Just forget all about it."

Then Lenny told Linda about the dead man in the cottage on the canal in Venice and about the movie set with the smiling posters of Gene McCarthy and the grim surprises of following the methaqualone trail. "That's not going to be us," he told her. "No fucking way."

Linda cried and buried her head in Lenny's neck while Daisy, the dog, tried to kiss them both. "Lenny," Linda said. "It's all going to be perfect, because I'm pregnant and now we can have the baby. I was afraid I was going to have to have an abortion."

Within an hour, Lenny and Linda were in the midst of packing. They were way behind on their rent, anyway, so they did not need to give notice, the way Lenny figured it. They hardly had any furniture left by then. The three-television home-entertainment complex was long gone. So was the top-of-the-line Sansui stereo. What was left properly belonged to Max. Anyway, it had terrible cigarette burns, so Max would probably just write it off and take a deduction. Their belongings were essentially what they had brought with them from New York, the dog, and a huge stack of American Express, Master Charge, and BankAmericard bills, all unpaid.

They began loading the car at ten in the morning. They had never gotten to know their neighbors—which is typical in Los Angeles—so that no one stopped to speak to them as they loaded their few things in Linda's Jaguar. Linda could not help contrasting their leave-taking with the way people had left her hometown in the Berkshires. When there was any hint of movement by a person or a family, everyone in town would gather to wish the traveler well. Now, an entire life had fallen apart and come to a close, and no one even said a word. Linda was glad they were leaving a place where people had no feelings for other people.

Lenny fought to keep himself from contrasting the departure from

Los Angeles with the arrival. Every time he started to feel crushed with disappointment, he thought of the body surrounded by Gene McCarthy posters in Venice. He might not be leaving as a prince of the city, but he was not leaving in a plastic body bag, either. Anyway, Lenny had a genius for rationalizing the inevitable. He told himself that he was not right for this L.A. place, anyway. He needed a place where it was quiet, where he could think and develop his ideas. You couldn't do that in a pressure cooker like L.A. It was for shallow, door-to-door salesmen, and not for people who think really big. Great ideas take time to germinate. They need a fertile soil, not freeway concrete. The saga of Lenny Brown was just beginning. This had just been testing him to see if he could understand the West. He understood it, even if it tricked him for a while. Now, he would withdraw from the fray and think about how to conquer.

Even as he looked through the house for anything valuable that he might have forgotten, while Frazier Smith played on the morning radio show over KLOS, Lenny could see himself as the sage of a small town, seeing the city from a distance, understanding it far better than anyone on the scene possibly could.

The protean Lenny could easily see himself remaking both himself and his image of himself. He was no longer the hustler, the schemer. Now, he was the Bernard Baruch of modern life, stepping off the treadmill to better grasp the essence of modern life and thereby subjugate it. Amazingly, miraculously, as Lenny thought about it, he no longer saw himself as a competitor with Joel or Michael or Max Sherman. He was the philosopher who had seen through the rat race. He could and did laugh at the people who were still in the maze. He loaded up his faithful Panasonic television which had been with him since college, which had patiently waited in a closet while he had the triple-decker, and which now worked perfectly as it always had. Yes, indeed, he thought, this is for me. The simple life with old, trusted, well-worn necessaries of life. No luxuries. No ostentation. Now, my mind is my pride and not my money, he thought. He actually started to laugh and sing to himself as he emptied out drawers and discarded the trinkets of his experiment in the rat race: packets of American Express bills, which he put in a closet next to other packets of bills; bowls of matches from La Scala, Matteo's, Mr. Chow, Ma Maison, Le Restaurant. My God, he thought, to think that this effluvia, this flotsam and jetsam of daily life, once meant anything to me! He threw away cans of liver paté; receipts from the Parisian Florist; automobile-repair receipts from Beverly Hills Mercedes; receipts from Carroll & Co., Men's Clothiers; check stubs for a hundred worthless checks. He packed the overdue notices from American Express in a hall closet.

He felt as if he were losing weight and gaining strength as every minute of packing went by. He paused in his work to take a shower. In the shower he began to sing about the amazing grace which had saved a wretch like him. To think he had once been blind and now could see! He was awakening from a trance. That was exactly it! Exactly! He had been a sleepwalker in a terrible nightmare, and now he was wide awake.

He had been dead, and now he was alive! Nothing less! He toweled himself dry and sang even louder. Amazing grace how sweet the sound! Which saved a wretch like me!

Before noon, Linda and Lenny had called the leasing company and told them to pick up their car. Lenny had called Marlys, told her he was leaving, that Max could have the house back, and that, "I don't hold a grudge against you for what you did. I had it coming to me. I hope you'll forgive me, too, for betraying the trust you had in me." Marlys was too shocked to reply.

Lenny left the door to the house wide open for the next suckers. At noon exactly they started up the car, with Daisy in the back seat, and headed for a new life in strict conformity with the fifty-five-mile-an-hour speed limit.

But where would they go? Lenny knew. Over a year before, he had gone to San José to scout out an industrial park. The local real-estate boys had taken him over the mountains for lunch to a small town called Santa Cruz. It lay in a crook in the California coast directly across the Monterey Bay from Monterey. Once it had been a fishing, artichoke, and mining town. Its streets still had Portuguese and Armenian names. Now, it was a major countercultural catchment, filled each year with a new crop of idealists because of its campus of the University of California. Its small Spanish-style houses, majestic mountains, dense redwood forests, and pervasive sea air had captured Lenny the moment he had seen the town from Highway Seventeen. On closer inspection, it was even more perfect.

It had beauty and it had peace.

Instead of the frenzy which was the fashion in Los Angeles, Santa Cruz positively reeked of calm and peace of mind. The townspeople seemingly prided themselves on their lack of concern with whether they got ahead, made money, or became famous. In Santa Cruz, the race was to the slow. The giant redwoods above the town did not care whether the man-insects made money or were broke. The ocean waves which pounded on the beach were utterly unconcerned with the price of stock or the availability of tax shelters. The fog which shrouded the town wrapped each person in a kind of visual insulation, so that each person might not be broken by the sights of a harsher, starker vision such as Los Angeles.

The town had come to Lenny's mind in dreams as a regular matter. It was a place of refuge for him, although he had never spent more than three hours in it. When the Jaguar edged onto the Golden State Freeway, it headed north, to Santa Cruz.

They did not take the scenic coast route which would have brought them past the glittering boys and girls of Malibu, because Lenny had no interest in such people any longer. They also did not take the route by the landed gentry of Santa Barbara, because what do such people know of struggle and deep thought? They avoided the Esalen Institute and Carmel, haunts of the idle rich, because what do the idle rich know of purification of the soul through suffering? What can a retired International Harvester dealer living on bonds have to say to a man and woman who have slogged through hell on their hands and knees, crawled on broken glass, hands cut and bleeding? Does Saint Sebastian talk to men and women in checked polyester trousers on a golf course?

Lenny and Linda roared through the central valley of California, the mighty San Joaquin, the world heartland of agriculture, a dusty, brown, bleached-out place with ugly low buildings with corrugated tin roofs and featureless drugstores and endless Harvestores. Their mood suited the purposeful, stark landscape, absolutely barren of style or artifice. In this place, and not in swimming pools, grew the stuff that counted: food and fiber. In Bakersfield and Fresno lived people who did things, not people who assumed postures. Thus, Lenny and Linda thought and spoke to each other during their trip through the San Joaquin crucible. By implication which did not need

to be verbalized, they were the kind of people who would also produce, without pretense or artifice. In the central valley, the food was
grown to feed the fools at La Scala. Lenny and Linda would now be
the nurturers, the growers of this world, not the parasites at restaurants with foreign names.

Although Lenny and Linda had not slept the night before, they
drove the entire distance, almost six hundred miles, in one day.
They stopped five times for gasoline, tacos, sodas, and rest. They felt
so happy from not being on Quaaludes any longer that they sang in
the car, something they had not done since they were dating and
drove out to Quogue once long before. That was in the days before
they knew how the world worked. Now they had seen the monster,
and they had escaped with their lives to sing and squeeze each
other's hands in love gestures all the way up a ten-lane road to a new
life.

When they got to the turnoff near Watsonville, it had been dark
for four hours. But neither of them felt tired. Daisy slept in the back
seat, but Lenny and Linda sang, "We ain't got a barrel of money,
maybe we're ragged and funny, but we're travelin' along, singin' a
song, side by side," and then sang songs from *Oklahoma*, which was
Linda's favorite.

What about the shark in Lenny's breast? I do not know. Perhaps it
had become frightened that Lenny would wind up like the man in
Venice. Then who would the shark have to gnaw upon? Perhaps
Lenny's revulsion and desperation at his situation had become so
great that he had grasped an oar and smashed the shark on the nose.
Perhaps the clever shark was simply biding its time. Or, finally,
perhaps the shark was so confused from the Quaaludes, the bad
checks, the scene in Venice, the scene at the tower in Century City,
that it was too dazed to attack. In its confusion, the shark might have
thought that Lenny was feeding it with accomplishment by as small
a thing as not killing himself with drugs.

Whatever the shark in Lenny felt, Lenny felt great. He had kicked
over the traces of drug addiction and a futile life. Now he was on his
way to a simpler, better way of living, changing the habits of his
entire adulthood. That move, from the Bloomingdale's in his envious
mind to J. C. Penney in a peaceful mind, was no small accomplishment.

From out of the Babylonian Captivity, across the parted Red Sea, into the land of milk and honey, across the River Jordan, Lenny and Linda, the wandering Jews or Italians or Czechs or whatever they were, headed up Route 1 to their deliverance. Just as they had once felt the anxiety fall off when they arrived in Los Angeles, so they could feel the anxiety melt away as they approached Santa Cruz. Once methaqualone had made them feel as if they would live forever. Now the road signs made them feel immortal. As they put each mile between them and Los Angeles, their lives became uncomplicated, simplified, *purified*.

Linda had an urge to ask Lenny to get off the road and kneel down next to him and give thanks to God. Blessed art thou, dear God, who makes us feel better. I often wonder if Lenny and Linda knew that they would be in very serious trouble for exactly as long as they judged each act not in terms of what it would accomplish, but in terms of whether it made them feel better.

By ten o'clock, Lenny and Linda pulled off the freeway onto River Street, the main street in Santa Cruz, a street of pancake restaurants, small bars, steak places with neon signs, and an immense modern courthouse which had genuinely fine architecture of stark concrete planes and broad windows behind even starker modern vertical concrete bars. There was hardly any traffic on River Street. Groups of children rode their bicycles along the sidewalks. There was no freeway noise. The air smelled of sea breezes. No crazy people ambled out from behind stores. In the distance, against the moonlit night sky, Linda made out the outline of the Ferris wheel at the Santa Cruz boardwalk. It was closed for the winter, but it still gave the skyline a festive, old-fashioned air.

There were no billboards.

There were little Spanish-style buildings and tiny one-bedroom bungalows off the main street. Palm trees grew in front yards. There were no Mercedes convertibles. There were also no knots of angry-looking Mexicans in lowered cars, daring Whitey to fight.

On several corners, there were ice-cream stands. Teenagers lined up neatly to get ice-cream cones under incandescent lights. There were no mercury-vapor high-crime lights.

Linda loved it so much that she cried in the car. She did not sob. Big, slow tears rolled down her face to show how incredibly relieved she was that she was going to have Lenny's baby in such a wonderful, cute, safe place.

They spent the first night at the Dream Inn, a plain cinderblock hotel right on the beach. Their room had a sliding glass window. They kept it open all night to hear the waves rolling and crashing. Lenny had to give the night man a dollar to sneak in Daisy. But before they went to sleep, the night porter, a thin, tall man wearing a bow tie, handed the dollar back under the door with a note: "A fellow lover of man's best friend."

Lenny and Linda slept peacefully that night and woke up the next morning feeling as if they had been born again in God's right hand.

The light in Santa Cruz was clear and bright. No pall of smog hung over the city. No doubt about it. Santa Cruz was the place for them. They ate a huge breakfast of sausages, eggs, orange juice, toast, apple slices, and coffee in a coffee shop overlooking the ocean. They were the only customers. The waitresses, all fat and pink, teased a busboy who was about to be inducted into the army.

After breakfast, they searched for an apartment. The first one they saw was perfect. It was in a small garden complex right near the ocean on West Cliff Drive. They did not have an ocean view in their particular unit, but as the manager pointed out, "People in this building are pretty considerate. If you really want to see the sunset, just go across the hall and there it is. A poet and his old lady live there. They love to have visitors." The manager had a potbelly and wore a tie. He was bald. When Lenny and Linda told him about Daisy, he rubbed his head and frowned. "I don't know about that," he said. "Let me see her."

The manager, Mr. Delmore, picked up Daisy and let her kiss his face. "I guess I couldn't keep out a cute little girl like her," he said. Daisy cried and squealed with happiness. Mr. Delmore said that they could sign the lease when they got around to it. He would like a two-hundred-dollar deposit for the dog, though, "Or else if the owners, some dentists from San José, hear about it, I'm back at the trailer court, and the missus would have my hide."

Lenny and Linda were moved in within an hour. Lenny carried in all the little boxes and the suitcases. Then, while Linda arranged their china and silverware and sang a song of her grandmother's, Lenny brought in his faithful Panasonic. He plugged it in and fiddled with the aerial while Linda wiped off the glasses and sang, "Then sings my soul, my Savior's God to Thee, how great Thou art . . ." Lenny tuned in the Monterey station. It was a special about the making of a star in Hollywood. There were scenes of the star looking for a two-million-dollar house in Beverly Hills. Linda walked over and turned it off. She gave Lenny a peck on the forehead, then went back to unpacking and cleaning the dishes.

"You did the right thing," Lenny said. "From now on, I just watch the football games."

He helped her unpack. Together, they sang songs from *Hair*.

Two days before, they had been Jack Lemmon and Lee Remick reeling in *The Days of Wine and Roses*. Now, they were in training to become "Ozzie and Harriet." When the baby came, they would be in "Father Knows Best."

Only those who have truly wallowed in self-hatred, lying dazed amidst cigarette ashes and Big Mac wrappers with an empty baggie once filled with Quaaludes and no idea of what time it is or what *day* it is, can really appreciate just how good it feels to be square.

The day Lenny and Linda took possession of the apartment on West Cliff Drive was a Saturday. They could not look for jobs until Monday. So they explored the town. They washed the Jaguar by hand, since they were not about to squander money on a car wash when they could do it themselves. They ate at a Taco Bell, because only fools need to eat at restaurants with French names. They drove up the Empire Grade into the densest redwoods Linda had ever seen. She had never even imagined that there were such dense forests somewhere near a major American city. For that matter, she was not exactly sure where they were, but that made the escape even more perfectly complete. They parked the Jaguar on an overlook and looked through a clearing in the redwood forest at the ocean. It shimmered and sparkled for a million miles out into space. It was as endless as Lenny and Linda's confidence that they were en route to a better life for them and their baby.

They had a cheeseburger at a stand in Felton, a tiny town tucked into a curve on Highway Nine, even more remote than Santa Cruz.

Every other eater at the stand was a biker or a biker's girl friend. They wore thick leather jackets and carried shiny chains. When Daisy jumped on the lap of a particularly tall one with no teeth,

Lenny tensed up. The biker held up Daisy, gave her a playful mock kiss, and carried her back to Lenny. "I love dogs," he said in a clear, precise accent. "They're better than people any day of the week."

That afternoon, Lenny and Linda walked through a forest behind the University of California. It went on forever. There was a carpet of pine needles two feet thick. Daisy kept tripping in it. In the middle of the afternoon, it was entirely in shade from the dense redwood trees. Lenny and Linda walked and talked and held hands and thanked God that they would be able to bring up their baby in a place where deer came up to you and sniffed at you and then walked away.

Amazing grace, how sweet the sound.

That night, for the first time since they had been married, Lenny and Linda left Daisy in the car and walked into an old stucco Presbyterian church on Bay Street. They sat in the pew nearest the back door, deep in their own thoughts. Then Linda knelt on the floor, even though it was out of place in a Presbyterian church. She thanked God that they had gotten out of hell.

Lenny and Linda were born for Santa Cruz. There was no better way to put it. From the first moment, it was fitted perfectly to their mood.

That saved a wretch like me.

When you are in a place which is suited perfectly to your state of mind, you get things done in a hurry, without the resistance which drains away joy. Within two hours, Lenny had found a job as manager of a small sporting-goods store on the Pacific Mall. The Mall was a three-block-long street of restored stores and cookie shops. Except for the hippie anachronisms lounging on the sidewalks, it was the cutest place Lenny and Linda had ever seen. There were two banks and ten cookie and ice-cream stores. There were no real-estate agencies and five clothing stores. There were even stores that sold used records, so that people from any economic background could afford good music.

Heinrich's Sports Shop was fifteen feet wide and about fifty feet deep. The owner was getting desperate when Lenny walked by and saw the sign saying, "Help Wanted." The last three managers had been more interested in closing down the shop and going hiking or surfing than in making sales. In Santa Cruz, people weren't really that into commerce. The manager of Heinrich's had to have at least a minimal commitment to keeping the place in business. The owner, Joe Heinrich, was getting to be about seventy, and if he didn't find a manager who could make the place work, he would just sell it and go out of business. The man had broken veins in his nose, but he still had all his teeth. "The wife says just close it down and let people go to Sears," Heinrich said. "But I like the idea that people will want to come to a place where someone remembers their names."

Lenny promised Joe (the owner insisted that Lenny call him Joe) that while he had not had much experience selling in the retail arena in the last few years, he had been pretty damned good at it in his youth and had even been the head of the men's department at Bloomingdale's. In the meantime, he had been in real estate, but that was a sucker's game. Too much pressure. Too little time with your family.

The owner said he understood where Lenny stood on wanting time with his family and would give Lenny a try, but he did want to know one thing: What was Bloomingdale's?

Linda found a job the same morning. By the kind of luck that had brought Lenny and Linda to Santa Cruz in the first place, the Office of Child Development had just received a grant of $311,000 for teaching of developmentally hearing-impaired children, which is to say children who were not born deaf but developed a hearing loss somewhere along the way, from trauma or virus, or causes unknown. The Office of Child Development had new offices on the top floor of the County Office Building facing the boardwalk, the Ferris wheel, and the ocean.

Helen, the head of the program (they did not use last names), was a hugely fat blond woman who wore polyester blue trousers just like the fat women you see in line ahead of you at supermarkets. She smoked constantly, virtually concealing her cigarettes behind the folds of fat in her palms. She wore harlequin sequined glasses which hung from the back of her head by a black string.

"You can really type seventy words a minute?" she asked.

"Yes, I can," Linda said. "I'll take the test anytime you say." Linda wore an Albert Nipon suit from the days when such things were important.

"Oh, hell, honey," Helen said, "you don't have to take the test. This is Federal money. Really, as long as you can put up with us, I guess we can put up with you."

Then Helen threw a spitball at a Mexican-American woman named Delores Bravo who sat across the office. Delores swatted the spitball away, then continued trying out different shades of nail polish on a sheet of typing paper which she yanked out of a Qantel word processor, causing a red light to start flashing on the sixteen-color data screen. Both women ignored the flashing red light. Delores said, "Sometimes Helen gets just a little raunchy."

"Me," Helen exclaimed, starting to laugh, setting off a virtual landslide of folds of flesh on her face. "What about that story you told me about you and those three cowboys at the El Dranel motel?"

"Oh, what about you and those guys from Lockheed in San José?" Delores said, tossing back another spitball.

"Anyway, we really do care about those deaf little kids," Helen said. "And someone who can type up the requests to get those kids money for tutors would really make a difference."

"Really," Delores Bravo added.

The job paid $240 a week, which was definitely top dollar for Santa Cruz. If Linda really needed the money ("like me," Helen laughed), she could start that very afternoon. Nobody else in Santa Cruz could type that fast, and that was for sure.

Lenny and Linda met back at the apartment for lunch. They ate peanut butter and jelly sandwiches. Who needed to show off any more? They talked about what a great place Santa Cruz was. They walked over and watched the seals at Lighthouse Point. They kissed each other as they sat on the grass and ate their sandwiches and Diet Dr. Pepper. Then Lenny told Linda that maybe she shouldn't eat anything with cyclamates while she was pregnant. She stroked his cheek with her hand and said, "That's why you'll make such a great father." Linda squeezed Lenny's hand. Three squeezes. *I love you.* Lenny squeezed back *I love you too.*

Linda went back to the County Office Building in the Jaguar. There was supergood bus transportation in Santa Cruz, so Lenny did not need the car. They were going to get by on one car, anyway, because why spend the money, and also, "Who needs to add more exhaust to a beautiful place like this?" Already, Lenny and Linda were feeling a sense of responsibility to protect this town and not just to exploit it, as they had felt about L.A.

Lenny took a bus up to the campus of the university and admired the concrete and redwood architecture. He marveled that the architects had been able to merge the soaring concrete and glass library so perfectly into the soaring redwood forest. He could not help contrasting it with the disgusting sprayed-stucco buildings in Los Angeles which he had sold to investors. Now he saw, with the artist's eye that was emerging from his forehead, which he had always suppressed until now, that he had genuinely assaulted the sensibilities of decent people with those buildings in L.A. Thank God he was gone from there, and in a place where beauty meant something to him and to everyone else.

At the library, Lenny browsed along the exhibit of pictures of seals and walruses. God, it was good to have the peace of mind to appreciate the grace of nature. As Lenny strolled through the library, he saw that day's *Wall Street Journal,* but he passed it up. Who wants to pick up anxiety on a printed page when you are in the midst of redwood splendor and azure skies?

As to the shark within Lenny, it, too, was mesmerized by the beauty of the place. Perhaps, the shark pondered, the arrival at such a place, the immersion in such beauty, was itself a sign of triumph and accomplishment. The shark, after all, had been on the prowl for many, many years inside Lenny's breast. Maybe it was now time for the shark to rest, too, and lose its hunger in the beauty of the redwoods and the shimmering ocean views.

That was how Lenny and Linda's new life began: Ocean seas shimmering and broken into millions of pieces, cloudless blue skies, and redwoods which laughed at the idea that there was anything in life more important than just taking in the beauty that God had given man for free. It began with the hope that by not asking too much, perhaps not too much would be taken away; and that by being thankful for the dawn of each day, engulfing hell would not devour Lenny and Linda's brains; and that by living without greed and ambition, life itself would take on a meaning beyond money and cars.

The job at Heinrich's was perfect. Kids came in with bleached blond hair and bought wet suits. Younger kids came in with their mothers and bought models of German cruisers. Girls came in to find presents for their boyfriends. Generally, Lenny recommended bicycles, if the girls could afford them, since bicycles were an ecologically sound way to travel, plus they built up the heart. If the girls could not afford bicycles, Lenny recommended model airplanes with tiny internal combustion engines. But he always cautioned the girls only to let their boyfriends fly them far away from houses so as not to ruin the day with noise pollution. He also sold rifles and shotguns, although he was opposed to hunting. It was not one man's place to tell another man how to live.

Lenny had one assistant, a thin, blond boy named Tim Mendes. The boy knew all there was to know about surfboards. Gradually, through Lenny's shrewdness at sales and Tim's knowledge of the boards, Heinrich's became the place for really serious surfers to come when they had saved enough to get a new board. Heinrich's was the first place in California to stock the new "Natural Progression" board made of textured polypropylene, which went through the waves like it had a mind of its own.

Sometimes in the morning the store was completely quiet. The kids were still in school. Tim worked part-time in the afternoons, when he was finished with surfing. The windows were tinted, and the sun came from a different direction in the morning, anyway. Sometimes Lenny sat on a plastic folding chair in the back of the store and looked over the rows of toys and models and tennis rackets and hockey pucks and roller skates and fishing reels, and Lenny thought. He thought that this dark, quiet place, surrounded by playthings, was exactly where he had wanted to be all his life. Something, parents or friends or magazine articles, had thrown him off course and made him try to be a hustler. What he really wanted was to be in a quiet place and think. Lenny told me that he felt more relaxed in that store in the mornings when no one came in than he had even when he took 'ludes. That is just how good being in the store made him feel.

Lenny had been thrown off course somewhere long ago. He had never intended to go out and compete with all the other boys. He wanted to have a few friends and then to be left alone. Was that too much to ask? In a world in which everyone was screaming for attention, why should anyone have bothered someone like Lenny, who wanted only to sit in a quiet, darkened room filled with toys? But someone had bothered him and sent him off to be thoroughly tormented in a twisted chase after what he never really wanted. That, at least, is a thought that often occurs to me about Lenny, after all that happened. Lenny wanted to sit by the seashore and watch the waves come in, to appreciate them and love their beauty. Someone convinced him that he had to wrestle with each and every wave. There was never much doubt after that as to who would win. But now Lenny had removed himself from the struggle and that was victory of a sort.

After Lenny had worked at Heinrich's for a few weeks, Tim suggested that they close up shop early on a certain drizzly Thursday afternoon. The two boys closed up, drove to Bonny Doon beach, ten miles north of town, and watched the nude swimmers. Tim told me later that Lenny did not even really notice the swimmers. He just looked at the waves. Tim said later that he thought Lenny cried, but Tim did not want to pry, so he did not look that hard.

A few days later, Tim bought Lenny a boogie board with his own money. It only cost twenty-nine dollars, but Lenny could not remember the last time someone had bought him a present just as a friendly gesture and not as a device to impress him or to put Lenny in his debt. Lenny gave Tim a case of Coors beer.

Pretty soon, Lenny and Tim began to spend Saturday afternoons together after the store closed at four. They would play tennis, or just watch a football game on TV, or drive up to Henry Cowell State Park and walk around in the redwoods. Tim was nine years younger than Lenny, but they still had a lot to talk about. Tim talked about how totally fucked the adult world was. "It's just like they put a plate of food in front of a bunch of starving wolves," he said, "and then told everyone that if you didn't get to the food, you were dead. But there's a lot of food around. There's not just one plate. That's a lot of crap."

Lenny told Tim that he had no idea how right he was. "It's a fucking jungle out there," Lenny said. "Just a fucking jungle. I can't tell you what it did to me. I was making a lot of money, and it still tore me up."

At first, Tim thought Lenny was bullshitting about how big a deal he was in L.A. But after a while, after many afternoons when Lenny and Tim had hoisted a few brewskis, Tim began to believe that

Lenny had really been a big shot, that something bad had happened, and that after that Lenny had decided to live a better, purer life. The thing that convinced him was that Lenny never initiated a conversation about the subject of money, and people who lied a lot usually began those conversations themselves. Tim had to admit that Lenny just might possibly be the kind of guy who would lead this country back to sanity, away from the mad craze for money. Plus, Lenny absolutely never touched drugs, which was very rare and impressive. Sometimes they would go over to the Catalyst to listen to a local band at the six o'clock "smoking hour," but even when everyone else in the place lit up, Lenny would stay with his Coors. He never got really abusive or loud. He just listened and occasionally put in a comment about how right the speaker was. He never said anyone was wrong. As far as Tim was concerned, Lenny was a very mellow guy.

Occasionally, Lenny got a little upset when men would come into the store and talk about big real-estate deals or stock deals or any kind of deals. Tim noticed that Lenny disliked grown men talking business in his store. Heinrich's was supposed to be for fun, and not for simply pursuing the chase after the buck. Lenny would sometimes get really red in the face when a big-shot real-estate guy walked in, Tim said, and would not wait on him unless he was not talking business.

For Lenny, the relationship with Tim was something more than he had bargained for. He could not remember the last time he had a male friend with whom he could talk and sit around in Lulu's or the Tea Cup without having to worry about impressing him or competing with him. It was really pretty great to have a buddy, a pal, to hang around with.

For Lenny, a male companion with whom he was not in an adversary posture was a godsend. Tim was no genius, but he was a friendly guy who never tried to make Lenny crazy. They would sit in the back of the store going over inventory on a Sunday morning, listening to KTOM, the Tall T from Salinas. The banter between them as they counted tennis rackets was music to Lenny's ears. Just having Tim call off the inventory-control numbers on the tennis balls was richly soothing to Lenny, like an incantation of friendly, peaceful spirits.

When Lenny told me about this, I tried to get him to tell me about his father and mother. Naturally, I would have expected him to have a passive father and a domineering mother to have gotten to the place in life where he found himself. But Lenny did not like to talk about his parents. When he did talk about them, he rarely said the same thing twice. Anyway, I am no psychiatrist, so we might just as well imagine what is most interesting to us. It is far too late to find out the truth now.

It is enough to know that Lenny had found that little corner of the world which is what everyone wants to find. You might call that place "safe," and you would be close to the truth. Or you might simply call it the place where Lenny could *rest*, and you would be close to the truth there, too.

Or you might say that Lenny had found a home.

Still, he got really upset when people came into Heinrich's and started talking about all the deals they had put together. He liked it best when he was completely alone in the store, or when just he and Tim were counting inventory.

Linda had never been as rootless as Lenny, and her Santa Cruz was not as nearly perfect. She talked with Delores Bravo and Helen about babies and about men. They ate their lunch at the McDonald's on Mission Street or out of a brown paper bag on the grass in front of the county building. Delores talked about how her boyfriend, Richard, a *huero*, was so fucked up on Maui Wowee that he regularly drove his truck into the window of his brother's house in Soquel. Helen talked about how she used to be really thin, like superthin, so thin that people would feel sorry for her, and really, she was happier now than she had been as a bag of bones with boys calling her "chicken legs."

Delores Bravo read *People* magazine out loud while the other two worked, like a replay of the ancient scenes on the lower East Side of New York, where cigar wrappers would be read to in Yiddish while they did their seamless work. Delores and Helen would always pause after they learned of a story about Suzanne Somers or John Travolta and ask breathlessly if Linda knew her or him. Linda never did.

"We used to hang around with people who had made a lot of money in real estate or car washes," she would say. "We didn't have much to do with the movie stars."

Once Delores read a story about an actress who had a ten-page split-beaver portfolio in *Penthouse,* then appeared, also nude, in a movie in which she played a nymphomaniac. She was interviewed in *People.* She said she would never in her life do anything which "was exploitative of myself."

Linda told Helen and Delores that the story summed up all of Los Angeles, as far as she was concerned. They did not get it.

Sometimes the county government subunits would hold parties for the girls who were leaving to get married or to have babies or to work on the Alaska pipeline, which had been finished for a few years, but no one told them. The parties would be at a small room off the main dining room, the Corsair Room, of the Holiday Inn. Invariably, the partygoers were all women. They left their husbands or boyfriends to watch TV or bowl while they hung around the Corsair Room, drank five margaritas each, and then told the dirtiest stories they could think of.

Linda had never heard women talk about sex with such attention to detail or in such crude terms as they did in the Corsair Room. She frankly thought that it was pretty disgusting. But she never stopped the girls when they talked about what big cocks black men have or never to get picked up by doctors because they can never get it up when they have to. She just listened and joked along with the others when the jokes got around to who was cheating on his expenses or who filed a request for Federal money that was twenty pages long and all the pages were blank. In the lives of Delores and Helen and their friends, this was the essence of humor, just as the size of black men's cocks compared with Mexicans' ("total losers in every way" was the general consensus) was the essence of relationships between men and women.

While Lenny walked in the redwoods with Tim or tried to achieve absolute quiet in the back room of Heinrich's, Linda grew restless. She had had enough of small town life back in western Massachusetts to last a lifetime. For Linda, New York had been the crowning glory of civilized man's achievements. Los Angeles had been fine when Lenny was doing well, although she had still preferred New York. She often said that she would rather live in New York poor than in Los Angeles rich. When she and Lenny fell into the Land of Nod, things deteriorated rapidly as far as Los Angeles was concerned. But when she dreamed of safe haven, she thought of the little apartment at Eighty-seventh and York.

Certainly, when she and Lenny had fled the body in Venice and the bills and the drug, she had been just as happy as Lenny. And certainly, she had been just as overwhelmed by the mountains and the redwoods and the shimmering seascape as Lenny. She had loved the simple life just as much as Lenny. She loved the new Lenny, the quiet, contemplative Lenny who only occasionally even glanced at the financial section of the newspaper. She was overjoyed to see Lenny happy. She and Lenny talked for hours about the kind of life they wanted for their child, and Linda would come close to tears with joy. To see Lenny alert, not obsessed, drugs totally gone from his system, was bliss for her and for Lenny.

But Lenny did not have to spend all day listening to a circus fat woman talk about the time she had taken on five black guys from a basketball team all at once in one room of the Dream Inn. And Lenny did not have to listen to a group of semiliterate women talking about their babies as if they wished the babies were dead. And finally, Lenny did not have to act nice to people who represented all the crudeness of small-town life that Linda thought she had left behind forever.

But while Linda was far from perfectly content, she was also far from as desperate as she had been only a few months before. Moreover, there was the baby to look forward to. If, in the terrible events which were soon to come, Linda had any secret motives of revenge against Lenny for bringing her to Santa Cruz or toward Lenny for keeping her on broken glass for a year and then putting her in a desert, that motivation was deeply buried under a large mountain of love for Lenny and for the child who was coming.

Still, even deeply buried forces can make a mountain move.

After Lenny and Linda had been incommunicado in Santa Cruz for about three months, lost to everyone but their parents back east, Lenny and Linda decided something. They were now secure enough in their new life so that they could get back in touch with some of the players in the most recent tragic act of their lives. After all, Joel and Rochelle were not completely bad people by any means. Joel had loaned Lenny money. Rochelle had always been a fan of Lenny's (although Linda knew nothing about the event in the pool house).

Through Rochelle, Linda had occasionally gotten involved in a charitable event of SHARE, with the other rich wives and girl friends in Beverly Hills. Perhaps Rochelle knew some better friends for Linda up in Santa Cruz. Perhaps Joel could accept Lenny as a philosopher and a friend, and not as a competitor or victim.

Lenny was extremely wary of picking up the phone and calling Beverly Hills. But Linda said that they would run into them sometime, anyway, just the way they kept seeing Jerry Brown in Los Angeles. They might as well be prepared.

When I think of Lenny and Linda calling Joel, I am reminded of the Japanese attack on Pearl Harbor. The most brilliant minds in Japan conceived the attack. They thought it would so dramatically humiliate America that America would withdraw from the central Pacific. One or two cautious voices asked what would happen if the attack did *not* make America pull out of the mid-Pacific but rather enraged us so much that we fought a total war. This question was considered extremely unpatriotic and was never, not even at the highest levels, addressed. After all, if the question had been seriously asked and answered, the attack would never have taken place. The only possible result of a war against the United States of America, a continental nation with an industrial and resource base perhaps one hundred times as large as Japan's, would be a Japanese defeat. Thus, a great catastrophe was *not* averted, simply because no one in power would follow a rash step to its most predictable consequences.

Lenny's call to Joel was his own attack on himself, with consequences which he probably glimpsed, but which Linda was so strongly determined to do that he shoved aside the knowledge of a certain eventual bad outcome and made the call, anyway. I often think that the anonymous man at the IRS almost killed Lenny with his plan on tax shelters and closing the loophole. Lenny recovered from that man and from himself, and moved to Santa Cruz. The telephone call to Joel was an entirely self-inflicted wound, although some might say that Linda, from whatever motivations she might have had, was cheerleading the hara-kiri show. In human life, causation is impossible to determine, and yet we all feel compelled to speculate. This is my speculation.

Linda convinced Lenny that he would feel even better about their stay in Santa Cruz if Lenny could show Joel just exactly what a fabulous place Santa Cruz was. Lenny said that he did not need Joel's approval to love Santa Cruz. Linda agreed entirely but thought that Lenny might just want to talk about old times. Lenny said the old times were terrible. Linda said that if Lenny felt that way about it, he certainly did not have to call. Naturally, Lenny then made the call.

Joel was delighted to hear from Lenny. He had heard all kinds of really strange rumors.

"If you take the worst of them, they probably weren't as bad as it was," Lenny said. "We were zombies."

"Ha!" Joel said. "I know you. It's all a smoke screen, and you're really building some giant development up there with Aetna. Right? A new city or something."

Even over the telephone, Lenny sighed. "Joel," he said, "you're a heck of a good pal. But I came up here not to even think about deals. So let's not even talk about deals or anything like deals. OK?"

Linda shivered when she heard Lenny talk. If he were that panicky about a few words about business, he was not as far from the Land of Nod as she had thought. She had the frigid feeling that she should never have encouraged Lenny to call Joel. She felt as if everything were slipping through her hands. She had that kind of sensitivity to situations. When Joel hinted that he was coming to Carmel and would be just a hop, skip, and jump away, Linda started to say into the extension that they would rather see Joel and Rochelle in L.A. someday. But it was too late. Lenny picked up the gambit.

"Come right over and see us. We're just in a really little place, but we'd love to see you. We can make a reservation for you at the Dream Inn."

After the telephone call, Linda told Lenny that she was really sorry that she had encouraged Lenny to call. "I want you to call him back tomorrow and tell him we're going east," she said.

"No way," Lenny said. "That would be too humiliating. After all, it was your idea to call."

Even now Linda occasionally tells me that if she had really insisted and had made certain that Joel did not come then or ever, they might still be living a small, peaceful life in Santa Cruz. But the past cannot be called back, as almost everyone knows. Lenny did not call back Joel. He had made his final appointment with fate and he planned to keep it.

Lenny went out after his conversation with Joel. He drove to the newstand on Pacific Street. He bought *Forbes*, the *Wall Street Journal*, and *Business Week*. The store was out of the *Institutional Investor*. He went to the store and let himself in. He went into the back room and began reading the latest business news. Tim happened to come in to see if Lenny might be there. Maybe Lenny wanted to go with him to watch the football game at a friend's house who had an Advent.

"Tim," Lenny said stonily, "pretty soon I'm going to have an Advent myself and a house big enough to put it in. I'm not going to be the manager of this little store forever. I have really big plans. In this world, you have to think big."

SANTA CRUZ, SUMMER 1979

VERTIGO

When I think of Lenny and Linda in Santa Cruz, escaping with their bare lives and then building a small Swiss watch of a life out of nothing, then inviting anguish into their lives, I often think of a poem by Hart Crane. The whole poem is far too long to include here, but it is basically about a man watching small children frolicking and playing on the beach. The narrator watches them in their youthful joy, and then he says, warned only by their superb happiness:

> O brilliant kids, frisk with your dog,
> Fondle your shells and sticks, bleached
> By time and the elements; but there is a line
> You must not cross nor ever trust beyond it
> Spry cordage of your bodies to caresses,
> Too lichen faithful from too wide a breast.
> The bottom of the sea is cruel.

The line for Lenny was getting back into the world where the shark held onto his heart so clearly. It was the boundary line separating where there is peace in a sporting-goods store on a quiet morning alone and the arena of struggle and competition and ostentation and absolute atomization of a continental peace of mind. The bottom of the sea is the end of everything, the place from where there is no return. Once, Lenny had been almost at the bottom of the sea, and he had returned. This time, with the call to Joel, he had added more than enough weight to keep himself down.

You may have wondered, by the way, how Lenny and Linda managed to take themselves off 'ludes so suddenly. The short answer is that I do not know how they did it. The longer answer is that the addiction of methaqualone, while genuinely physical, has a powerful psychic connection. The body craves the drug to smother receptors in the brain. Apparently that has been proved in laboratories. But the receptors of the brain can be soothed by secretions from the brain itself, called prostaglandins. These fluids can be secreted by administering electrical shock to the Quaalude addict. Somehow, the jolt makes the brain produce its own opiates, which replace the missing methaqualone.

In the case of Lenny and Linda Brown, the shock of realizing how close they were to being the dead man in the cottage in Venice was all the shock they needed. Lenny had two 'ludes on the way home from the beach. But after that, when he saw his wife and realized that they could someday be dead simply from seeking to buy Quaaludes, their own brain fluids took over.

Moreover, when the brain is happy, it also secretes substances which the receptors crave. For those first few days in Santa Cruz, their cortexes were producing prostaglandins faster than Nissan makes Datsuns. By the end of a week, the receptors got accustomed to not having their methaqualone and instead looked to the brain's secretions. Since Lenny and Linda were doing new things, laughing on Twin Lakes State Beach with Daisy scampering behind, their receptors picked up all that they needed from their brains. After that, there was only a residual psychological craving, which Lenny and Linda overcame by talking about their future and the unspoken knowledge that drugs can make a baby *in utero* come out like Billy Carter.

For this medical knowledge, I am indebted to Barbara Bernstein, M.D., the only real name in this book.

To put Lenny and Linda's withdrawal another way, imagine that they were told that they would be put before a firing squad if they took 'ludes and that they would live forever if they didn't. Even a real physical addiction can be beaten with such a combination of incentives (and if it cannot, then why are people ever able to lose weight on diets?).

Lenny and Linda had stepped far away from Hart Crane's line on Quaaludes. Linda, therefore, assumed they were safe. She had not then understood (although she does now), that the Quaaludes were the outer manifestation of the inner anguish that being in the jungle of total competitiveness meant for Lenny. The Quaaludes themselves were no more the danger than uranium in a mine is the danger. They were mere instruments through which the madness of a man never made for combat but thrown into daily battle was turned upon himself.

Now we pick up Lenny and Linda one short week after the conversation with Joel. Linda is at home doing needlepoint and watching a rerun of "The Avengers." She can hear the surf breaking across West Cliff Drive. She looks extremely pregnant in her expectant mother's outfit of large jeans and a floppy shirt. While she waits for Lenny to come home, she constantly looks at her Timex watch (she sold the Gerard Peregeaux long before, in return for one hundred genuine Rohrer 714's). At eight o'clock, Joel and Rochelle are expected. Linda hopes that by dressing up as even more pregnant than she is, she can and will move Joel to have pity on Lenny and not make him and her crazy with talks about deals and money. She has planned that they will go out for a quick cheap dinner at the Taxco Gardens. Then she will send Joel and Rochelle back to their world. She, Linda, will be extremely glad to be in the boring world of Helen and Delores Bravo again if she can just keep Joel from making Lenny totally insane.

The problem is that the impending visit of Joel and Rochelle has made Linda extremely nervous. Not just a little twinge of care here and there, but a deep, permeating edge of terror is eating into her body. Not only has Lenny changed dramatically for the worse since the call to Joel, but there is every evidence that he is poised for a long dive. For the last week, he has been unable to sleep past six in the morning. He gets up early, goes in to the Dean Witter office across from Long's Drugs, and has long, fantastic talks with Eric Smythe, a broker there. Linda knows that the talks are totally fantastic because occasionally Eric calls and leaves a message about buying

$160,000 worth of Reynolds Metals or 210,000 shares of Columbia Pictures at twenty-one dollars a share.

At the time, Lenny and Linda, by careful saving, have $1,373 in their savings account.

Linda then waits by the faithful Panasonic, doing needlepoint, so nervous that her hands are trembling. Finally she has to stop doing the needlepoint and have a small glass of chablis, which will probably do the baby a lot more good than being so nervous, which can also hurt a fetus. The wine is not nearly enough, though. She knows what would be enough.

Meanwhile, where the hell is Lenny? If only he were in the apartment and Linda could talk to him, squeeze his hand with the *I love you* message, she might be able to keep him from going over the brink.

But Lenny is not at the apartment on West Cliff Drive. He is at the track down below Cowell College at U.C. Santa Cruz. It is a wide, grassy plain with a stupefying view of the Pacific. Many brokers and land speculators go there at the end of the day to run off the craziness of the work. Lenny has begun to go there, too. In Santa Cruz, everyone knows everyone else. All the brokers from the University of Santa Clara know that Lenny is the manager of Heinrich's sporting-goods store. But Lenny has dropped a few hints about sisters who know Jackie Onassis and a mother who jumps horses and a crazy inventor father. So the word gets around pretty quickly. Lenny Brown has got family money, the best kind to have. He is in a job which gives him time to play, but if the right deal came along, Lenny Brown has got the horses back east with his family and their crazy fox-hunting friends.

On this night, when Linda waits with trembling hands, Lenny jogs next to Raul Seitz, whose family owns a small department store. Raul is a young guy who owns a small brokerage in Capitola. He has a big chin and a wide face and short hair. He looks like a casting director's dream of a rich man in his early thirties in a California coastal town. He and Lenny talked about a possible straddle in soybeans and soybean oil, known as the "soybean crush," in which you make your money by going short against the bean and long on the oil, or maybe I have it backward. Lenny had to be really briefed before he saw Joel. He wanted Joel to think he was laid back, but he also wanted to let Joel know that he, Lenny, knew exactly what was happening in the world of deals.

Raul Seitz later told me that Lenny listened attentively, asked smart questions about how the spread would be affected by commissions, and then saw a poor lost Golden Labrador. Lenny stopped talking about tenths of a cent, stopped jogging, and walked directly over to the Labrador.

The dog was wet. It had a cut on its nose. It cried when Lenny came near to it, but it did not run away. Lenny had that effect on dogs. He might not have been able to overturn the power of the IRS, the *Wall Street Journal,* and even the self-destructive demons within his soul. But he had a rapport with dogs which only a few lucky people ever have. They knew he was serious. Lenny began to pat the dog. It was shivering. He hugged the dog. It was cold.

Lenny told Raul that he would have to finish up on the straddles later. "But it's a fantastic concept," he said. "Sort of like gambling, but without the risk." Which is exactly the way Raul Seitz had been searching for to explain it to his clients. He made a mental note to offer Lenny a job as a registered rep at his brokerage. Lenny told Raul he would have to take the dog to a vet and get that cut taken care of, and then maybe find someplace to stash the hound until he could find it a good home.

It was time for Lenny to drive down Bay Street and meet Joel and Rochelle. But he decided he could be a few minutes late. He put the dog into the Jaguar and drove it to a twenty-four-hour vet he knew on Forty-first Street in Capitola. Then he talked to the vet for a few minutes about where he might keep the dog so that it would be safe and sound and would not, under any circumstances, be put to sleep or used for experiments. Lenny hated even to think of animals being used for experiments. The idea that people just tortured animals to death to get research grants, that they put ground glass in puppies' eyes to get a few bucks from a foundation, sometimes made him think of committing murder.

The vet suggested that Lenny bring the poor shivering Labrador to a woman named Sheryl on Branciforte Drive. The woman was as opposed to medical experiments on animals as Lenny was. She would keep the dog for as long as it took to find a good home if Lenny paid for the board, which would be only a few dollars a week. Lenny thanked Bernie Goldsmith, the vet, and went off to find

Sheryl. He knew that Joel and Rochelle were there by now at his apartment. But he also knew that Linda was a goddam sight more eager to see them than he was and also that Linda loved dogs, too, so that she would understand if he took another few minutes to find a poor innocent lost Labrador a home.

Sheryl Van Dam was a young, short, busty woman with a big smile and sad eyes. She looked at the Lab, then at Lenny, and she said, "You must be a saintly man to do this for a dog you don't even know. Please come in for just a few minutes."

The woman had a two-bedroom house which looked as if it had come right out of a James M. Cain novel. It had a living room of about twelve by fifteen feet with one sofa, a chair with burst springs, and portraits of Martin Luther King, Jr., Bobby Kennedy, and John F. Kennedy, although the woman was undeniably white and even said that she had gone to Miss Porter's school in Farmington, Connecticut. She had the portraits up, she said, to remind her of how persecuted people must feel all over the world. "And that's the closest I can come to understanding how a dog must feel that only gives out love and affection, and never does anything bad, and people treat it as if it were just there to be tortured." The woman smoked Viceroys, just like Lenny, and had once been in the trainee program of the Morgan Guaranty Trust Company. She wore a Villager sweater and a gold circle pin, but the sweater had holes in the elbows and the gold circle pin had somehow become rusted.

She wanted to know all about what a saintly man like Lenny was doing in Santa Cruz. She wanted to introduce Lenny to all twelve of her dogs. "The landlord used to complain all the time," she said, "so I finally got so sick of it that I called my trustee in Boston and had him buy the damned place."

By now, Lenny was an hour and a half late for his rendezvous with catastrophe. He knew that it was time for him to get home. It made a good impression on people to keep them waiting, as if you had more important things to do. But he also knew that it was a sure thing that Linda would be really pissed if he were much later. He turned down the offer of a glass of Cribari Brothers Mountain Burgundy in a Baccarat glass with a spider's web inside. He thanked Sheryl, took her phone number, and headed home. Sheryl Van Dam remembers that Lenny looked as if he would rather stay and talk about dogs. "I have some people at my house," he said, "and I guess I have to see them, even though I really can't stand to be in the same room with them. My wife likes them, though."

Sheryl was really surprised when Lenny mentioned that he was married. She figured that he was going to try to fuck her, for sure, and frankly, she thought he was a kind of sensitive guy, the kind you don't see much of in Santa Cruz. "I wish he had stayed, to tell you the truth," she said. "I could have made him earn his keep," she added with a wink. She had light blue eyes. She was already drinking straight scotch at ten A.M. when I met her.

Lenny turned the radio in the Jaguar to KTOM, the Tall T in Salinas, and drove down the highway of fate. But, as usually happens, fate had already dealt Lenny's hand and left it lying on the table in the cute apartment on West Cliff Drive. The cards were waiting for Lenny to pick them up. Then he could weep. The highway turned out to have nothing to do with it.

Back at the apartment, two hours before, Joel and Rochelle had pulled up in a black Porsche 911, completely restored to Concours condition, with a slight change. Joel had had the Becker Mexico taken out and a digital Nakamichi cassette deck put in. He was listening to the "Ride of the Valkyries" from the *Niebelungenlied*, as he pulled up. Linda remembers hearing it through the open door.

Daisy barked, and Joel and Rochelle and Linda hugged each other. Joel looked unusually respectable. He wore a leather vest, corduroy trousers, and a normal shirt with no chains or bracelets. Rochelle wore baggy jeans, which were just starting to be featured in *Vogue*'s advertisements. Her hair was much shorter than it had been. She still had her tiny, perfect features, but her mouth was permanently half open now, as if she might bite someone if she got bored.

They drank Mouton Cadet wine, which Joel had brought four bottles of, and they talked about how pregnant Linda looked and how relaxed she looked. Joel said that if he had had any idea of just how deeply Lenny and Linda had been suffering from Quaaludes and from money problems, he would have gotten them into Tecate for a rest cure pretty damned quick, and he would have gotten Lenny a job so he shouldn't have to walk around carrying that kind of weight all day long. "That's just not right for a nice guy like Lenny," Joel said.

Rochelle felt like saying that Joel was a total liar, because, after all, Joel had really gotten off on lording it over Lenny and getting her and Lenny jacked up on 'ludes so that they started to make out in front of him. But she did not say anything, because after all, Joel had just started in psychotherapy with a fairly heavy hitter in the shrink world, and maybe Joel needed help and not a reminder of what a total putz he was.

They talked about what a completely crazy place Los Angeles was, and how, particularly at this time of year, the smog was so bad that you could hardly believe it. "When I take off out of LAX," Rochelle said, "it looks like we're flying out of the inside of a vacuum-cleaner bag. That's the truth." She smoked Marlboros nonstop, which was new. Linda thought maybe she should tell Rochelle to lay off, because ambient smoke was not good for babies, but Rochelle had just gotten there and Linda did not want to start acting like a maniac.

Joel talked about how much he loved hearing the sound of waves and that he really hoped that when he got back to L.A., he could find the time to look for a little place in the Colony, maybe like the place Lenny and Linda once had. "By the way," Joel asked, "did you rent that place or buy it?"

Rochelle said, "Shut up, Joel. We didn't come here to play those games."

Joel said, "I was just asking."

They talked about the schools in Santa Cruz, and Joel started to fidget with a box of matches from Mr. Chow.

Linda began to get seriously worried about Lenny. He was usually the promptest guy on the block. If he were late, that would not be too surprising—at any rate if he were only a few minutes late—because Linda knew he was dreading this visit. But he was over half an hour late. Linda began to tremble. Her voice began to quaver. She did not know why she was quite this nervous. Partly it was her thought that if something had happened to Lenny, she would kill herself. Partly it was her fear that she had dragged Lenny into a meeting that was going to completely undo him mentally, as he threw himself back into the machinery where Joel was so comfortable and where he was so scared. For these reasons and because she was a sensitive, frightened person, Linda began to shake.

Joel saw her trembling and said, "We each took a half a 'lude before we got here. It common denominators you out, and it doesn't make you high or anything. It's just like taking a mild tranquilizer."

"I'm pregnant," Linda said. "No drugs."

"Linda," Joel laughed, "half a 'lude is like having one glass of wine. I think you'd probably be better off with half a 'lude than with wine, anyway."

Rochelle said, "I think he's right. Half a 'lude this late in your pregnancy can't make that much difference."

Linda thought about it. She was so nervous by now, so completely terrified that Lenny might have had an accident, that Lenny might even have left her for having dragged Joel back into his life, so generally alone in this miserable apartment in a miserable part of the world, without any friends except Helen and Delores Bravo, that she giggled and reached out her open palm. Joel put four 'ludes in it. "Some for later," he said. "For when you have the baby and can't sleep."

Linda went to the sink and poured water into a cup. She swallowed two 'ludes before she even remembered that she was supposed to take only half of one.

As soon as she realized what she had done, she felt as if she had unleashed all the demons of hell upon an unsuspecting world. She had an instant in which to see all of her life that had come before, the farm in the Berkshires, the life in New York, the nightmare in L.A., and the abyss that now yawned in front of her, bottomless, insatiable, ineluctable. Good-bye, she thought, good-bye and good-bye and good-bye. In some way, standing at the sink with its Formica counter of bright yellow, holding a white plastic coffee cup filled with water, she realized that she had now made a break with everything that had come before and started on a path to somewhere completely uncharted and frightening. She had, in a sense, renounced her faith, although she had only an instinctual realization of that at the moment she swallowed the 'ludes. She felt terrified.

She sat down heavily in the kitchen, which was part of the living room. Rochelle said Linda looked as white as a sheet. Rochelle said she and Linda and Joel should walk by the beach. Linda felt that the walls were closing in on her. She was happy to get out to some spot where she might escape what she had done and seen, mocking her, her whole idea of a future, in that little apartment.

Now that it is all over, I often wake up in the middle of the night and wonder how Linda could have taken those 'ludes and thrown away her grasp on the future (or, as it happened, Lenny's future).

She was not a bad or mean person. Far from it. She was not a spiteful woman. She genuinely loved Lenny and wanted them to succeed. At the very least, she wanted some measure of peace of mind, which is what we all want. At four A.M., I look at the lights of L.A. and wonder what could have made her take the Quaaludes and voluntarily step before the firing squad of life's horrors. I have no answer except that when IBM designs the computer that can answer all questions, if that computer is as smart as IBM will say it is, if you program in the story of Lenny and Linda, the computer will print out tears.

Linda and Joel and Rochelle and Daisy walked slowly down the stairs to the ground. They walked slowly because, if the truth be known, Linda was not the only one who had taken two 'ludes. Rochelle and Joel had taken at least two themselves. The night was going to be a strain for them, too, after all. As usual in Santa Cruz, there was a heavy fog covering everything. Linda led the way to the beach, because she had walked it so often that she knew the way across the grass and down to the beach by heart.

Daisy walked a few feet in front, as if to earn some small part of her Alpo by seeing into the fog. There was almost no traffic on West Cliff Drive, so the adventurers were able to cross the street safely to the thin margin of grass which marked the top of a cliff over the steep hill which led down to the beach. There was a powerful tide that night, as there is almost every night. Linda could hear the pounding of the surf upon the sand, as if it were calling her personally to account for a tragedy she knew would come. But the sand did not answer the waves, and so Linda had no idea what the punishment meted out to her might be.

Joel said, "I'd like to go down to the beach. That way I could tell everybody back in town that I went into the ocean at night, and that would really blow them away."

Rochelle said, "Fuck you, Joel. It's too steep. If you want to go, Linda and I'll wait up here."

Linda said, "It's not really that steep if you know the way. There's a little stairway almost that the surfers have carved out."

She began to walk down the small stairway. It was more like a slippery steep path, lubricated with the wet air of a seashore evening. After a few feet, you might have seen a wooden board containing the elementary rules of surfing. "Paddle around waves, not through them." "First surfer on board has right of way." And a few others that I no longer recall.

Daisy walked a few feet ahead once again. Joel walked behind in his Gucci suede slippers, looking for all the world like a Hasid about to go surfing.

Linda turned around after a few feet to see if Joel was still behind her. He was, and so she turned back and kept walking. That was when she tripped over an old rubber flipper that a surfer had left in the path. She reached out for something to steady her. There was nothing, so she slid backward, then pitched forward and then fell head over heels down the side of the path, over a small cliff, and down to the large, flat, hard rock, which she hit with her belly.

Joel started to shout to her to ask if she were all right. Rochelle ran down the path like a comet. She examined Linda, then ran up the path in her high-heeled pumps, and ran across the street to a monastery dormitory. She smashed in the glass door and opened the handle. Then she picked up the first telephone she saw and called the operator. She described just where she was, described the accident, then ran back across the street to Linda, who was now conscious but was crying and moaning like a creature from a forest trapped in a cruel steel clamp.

The paramedics were there in fifteen minutes. They had been rescuing a skateboarder with a broken ankle. Linda was in the operating room of the New Dominican Hospital on Soquel ten minutes after that. Three hours later, in the recovery room, they told her that she had internal bleeding, which they had controlled with surgery, contusions about the head and arms, and a concussion in her brain. The baby, they added, was completely lost, but apparently she was not hurt so badly that she could not have others. The blood screen had turned up a high level of methaqualone, Dr. Bernbaum told her, which might teach her a lesson about how human mothers should act in this world. He had seen so many women who thought they didn't owe their babies a thing that he sometimes thought he would move to a cabin in the woods and just read Jane Austen. He obviously did not know much about Jane Austen if he thought he would find mothers who were truly devoted to their children in her books, but the point was made as far as he was concerned.

To Linda, the point had been made the moment she felt herself falling on the path. The point might even have been made the moment she realized that she had taken two Quaaludes. Anyway, the real point was now a few pounds of dead, twisted tissue in a stainless-steel tube leading away from the hospital and into eternity. Linda did not need any examples from Jane Austen.

She did need the visit from Lenny. He had gotten to the hospital just as Rochelle and Joel were about to leave to look for him. Santa Cruz is a small town. The word had gotten around West Cliff Drive in a hurry. By the time Lenny had left Sheryl Van Dam's house, arrived home, and fortified himself to confront Joel, there was the landlord, with his cardigan sweater, sitting in the kitchen nook.

"There's been an accident," he said. "Linda fell down a path near the beach. She's at Dominican."

Lenny saw the black Porsche in the parking lot.

He rushed over to the hospital. He ran twelve straight red lights. He got to the waiting room and saw Joel looking sweaty and pale. Joel began to hug him, man-to-man style, to reassure him. Lenny pushed him away.

Rochelle explained what happened. "It was our fault," Rochelle said. "We shouldn't have let her take us for a walk at night. It was crazy."

"We didn't force her to take the 'ludes," Joel said. "She asked for them. We figured she could still handle them."

Like a suddenly released coiled spring, Lenny whirled around toward Joel. He hit Joel in the stomach with his fist as hard as he could. Then he hit Joel in the side of the head as hard as he could. Joel was on the floor amidst a pile of *Reader's Digest* and *People* magazines. The nurse on duty in the waiting room did not look up from her copy of *TV Guide*. Rochelle helped Joel up. She looked at Lenny as if to say, "I don't blame you."

Then she and Joel went outside to wait for a taxi. They had gotten to the hospital with the paramedics.

Lenny had to wait about an hour before he could see Linda. Then he saw Dr. Bernbaum coming out of her room. Dr. Bernbaum, a fat man with tiny hands and a mustache and a generally finicky air, told Lenny that he was lucky that his wife was alive. "Quaaludes and babies don't mix," he said. "Next time you want to have a baby, you'd better decide between the baby and the Quaaludes."

In a tiny room Linda lay on her side, crying and moaning, rocking back and forth, hugging herself, shaking with sorrow and madness. There was a large cruciform above her on the wall, with a Christ in such vivid torment that he might have been able to understand just what Linda was going through.

Lenny sat down lightly next to Linda and said, "No matter what, I'll always love you. Always. I know it wasn't your fault. We'll always have each other and it'll be all right. We'll have another baby and we'll be all right."

He told her that for about two hours, stroking her hair and kissing her as he talked. She just cried and held his hand and pressed it against her forehead. After two hours, a black nurse came in and told Lenny he had to leave. Lenny kissed Linda, squeezed her hand in their code, then left. Joel and Rochelle were gone from the waiting room as he passed through it.

Lenny drove home without listening to the radio. When he arrived, he looked out the window for a long time. Daisy had come home and sat on the porch, waiting for Linda. She would not come in, even when Lenny offered her a dog biscuit.

At about midnight, he drove to a liquor store on Mission Street. He gave José, the night manager, fifty dollars. José gave him seven 'ludes. They were real ones, not boots. Lenny took three when he got home. The next morning, he took three more. The next afternoon, he went out to the bank, cashed a check for two hundred dollars, then bought thirty more 'ludes. He did not leave the apartment for two days. When Linda was released from the hospital, she had to take a taxi home. She understood what had happened.

Lenny had already called Joe Heinrich and quit his job. He had also called Delores Bravo and told her Linda was quitting. "We have an incredible opportunity in real estate in L.A.," he told her. That is what he told Joe Heinrich, too.

He called me in Los Angeles and told me that something terrible had happened. He laid out the whole story. He cried over the telephone for a long time. I could hear a rerun of "Star Trek" in the background. "I can't understand how it could have happened," he said ten times. "Things were going so well. Really, so goddam well."

Then he said that if his life were going to be totally out of control, he might as well make some money while he was at it. So he was coming down to Los Angeles to make a real killing in real estate.

"No working for someone else this time. That's the fool's way out. This time I control the money. I'm the boss."

He also told me that he had heard about a small French restaurant in Encino where the food was better than at L'Ermitage and the prices were a lot lower, but you had to be a friend of the maitre d' to get a table. "Luckily, I met him up here," Lenny said, "so we're all set when we get to Los Angeles."

Linda rested and packed for three days. She hardly spoke the whole time. Lenny was wrecked on 'ludes most of the day, anyway, and when he wasn't, he frantically read the *Wall Street Journal*. Linda tried to tell him how sorry she was. He would shrug and say, "That's life. Things are tough for everybody." Then he would go back to the *Wall Street Journal*.

Ten days after Linda lost the baby, Lenny and Linda sold the Jaguar for three thousand dollars. That was not much of a price, but the car had quite a few scratches by then. Also, of course, they did not really own it and had to swear falsely on an affidavit that they did. It really belonged to Southwest Leasing in Beverly Hills, but Southwest would never miss it. After all, they had insurance. So Lenny and Linda sold it for three thousand. They bought a used Subaru for two thousand. It was dark blue and really, Lenny said, ran better than the Jaguar. That was Japanese industrial efficiency at work, Lenny explained. They bought seventy-five Quaaludes with five hundred dollars from José. About a third were boots, but the others were real Lemmons, right off the truck, as José said with a smile. Then they said good-bye to the landlord and to Tim and to Joe Heinrich and to Delores and Helen. Lenny sent a check for fifty dollars to Sheryl for the care of the golden Lab. They put Daisy in the car and left just as the sun came up over the mountains and broke the gray sea into a million, billion shifting planes and lights, just as the sea air was beginning to smell really sweet. They turned on the car, each took a 'lude with Diet Pepsi, and they headed back toward Los Angeles, the way a dead spirit walks back into its grave at morning.

DEPORTEES

Connecting nothing with nothing: A journal of Lenny and Linda's return to Los Angeles. First of all, there was no limousine at the airport and no jovial man in a cowboy hat. Instead, there was the 1971 Subaru wheezing into town in the middle of the night, almost out of gas, steam rising from the hood, one tire so bald the fabric showed through. The first night, they slept in the car in Poinsettia Park in the worst part of Hollywood, surrounded by winos and homosexuals. The back seat was crowded with cardboard boxes, so Lenny and Linda took turns sleeping in the front seat while the other read the classifieds for an apartment. The next morning they washed up in a Denny's on Sunset, then started searching. What they needed was not easy to find: an apartment which was supercheap, which would take a dog, and which did not require any money in advance. Lenny and Linda had about five hundred dollars, but they needed to save that to set Lenny up in his own real-estate consulting business. After all, Lenny had returned to Los Angeles to take the town by storm with his newfound knowledge of just how tricky everything was. The last time he had been a sucker, but this time he was wise. Their apartment could be very humble, because Lenny would be spending most of his time at his office, setting up deals.

That first morning, after several cups of coffee at Denny's, Lenny and Linda drove east on Hollywood Boulevard. Lenny looked at the

apartment buildings on the right side of the street. Linda was re-
sponsible for the buildings on the left. The dirty windows of the
Subaru made the horrible group of buildings look even more horrible, if that was possible. The temperature gauge in the Subaru kept
going up. By the time they got to La Brea, the car had overheated.
They had to stop at the self-service Shell station for water.

Lenny and Linda were poor, but certainly not destitute. Why,
then, did they sleep in the car, wash at Denny's, and act like bums?
Because they now thought of themselves as bums, pure and simple.

Linda told me later that: "I could see that the idea of living in one
of those slum buildings on Hollywood was driving Lenny crazy. It
was driving both of us crazy, I guess." While they waited at the gas
station for the Subaru to cool, Lenny took a Quaalude. "He was kind
of secretive about it," Linda recalled, "but not so secretive that I
wasn't able to catch him taking the pill. When he saw I was looking,
he asked me if I wanted to split it with him. There was no point in
saying that I did. He had already swallowed it."

It was quiet in the Subaru as they drove up La Brea to Franklin. As
they made a left turn on Franklin, Linda spotted a For Rent sign
outside of a building on the corner. She told Lenny to stop the car.
Lenny pulled over and just sat behind the wheel. He stared into the
middle distance and did not say a word. "Come on," Linda said as
she moved to get out of the Subaru. "Lenny, we should check this
out. Don't you want to look at the apartment?"

The building was called the Hamilton Arms. Lenny did not need
to look at the apartment because he had been there before. He had
scored 'ludes at the Hamilton Arms many times in those last two
dark months in Los Angeles before they went to Santa Cruz. His
connection at the Hamilton Arms had been an aging alcoholic who
had stolen a bunch of Quaaludes from his brother's drugstore in
Pasadena and who was willing to sell them for ten dollars apiece.
The connection's name was Mel. Mel was able to steal Quaaludes
from his brother's store, Mel had bragged to Lenny, because Mel
knew when his brother, a dying man, had to leave the store for
chemotherapy sessions. Mel's apartment was even filthier than Bob
Thornton's. Lenny had often postponed a trip to the Hamilton Arms
until he was physically sick from lack of methaqualone. He hated
the Hamilton Arms. Lenny told Linda to get back in the car. He told

her that they could do better. The thought of Linda living in a place like the Hamilton Arms made a lump churn in Lenny's stomach. Linda closed the door. Lenny put the idling Subaru in gear and headed west on Franklin.

"Lenny told me he thought that with a little luck and some of his famous fast talking, we might be able to get a place in Laurel Canyon," Linda said later. "We didn't fool ourselves. We knew we couldn't afford anything fancy. Not this time. Maybe just one bedroom, maybe a little yard. Maybe a little apartment."

The cute little one-bedroom houses in Laurel Canyon started at $650 per month. The apartments, like the ones on Honey Drive, the wooden complex originally built by Louis B. Mayer in the 1920s to house homeless MGM starlets, were a little cheaper, but not much. Even the smallest shoebox cost $450, and the people wanted first and last month's rent plus a hefty security deposit. And that was if Lenny and Linda could find one available for rent. That first afternoon, guided by a hand-printed sign at the Country Store, the Canyon community market, they were shown a tiny apartment above a redwood cabin.They were almost able to rent it.

The apartment was owned by a young black man in his mid-twenties who spoke with a soft African accent. Lenny talked big: He told the landlord that he was in the real-estate business himself, was just getting started in Los Angeles, and that money would be forthcoming from his office in Santa Cruz. Linda did not like the way Lenny stretched the truth, but sometimes that was the only way to deal with these landlords. After all, they were back in Hollywood, where everyone loved a good story.

Lenny talked the man down to $350 per month, knocking one hundred dollars off the price in exchange for taking care of the complex's small garden area. "Hell," Lenny said, "watering plants relaxes me, takes my mind off business. And it looks like those plants need some taking care of." Linda nodded agreement. Then Lenny brought up the subject of their dog.

The landlord loved dogs. He thought every family should have a dog. He wanted to meet Lenny and Linda's dog. Lenny and Linda took the landlord out to the double-parked and steaming Subaru and let Daisy out of the stuffy, strangling car air. Daisy was perfect. She sat when Lenny said "Sit" and shook hands with the landlord upon command. The landlord let Daisy lick his hand, and he patted her on the head. Lenny and Linda smiled at each other. The landlord loved Daisy. He even said so. Then the landlord said that the dog could stay if Lenny paid a $500 cleaning deposit before they moved in. He said he would hold the place for twenty-four hours, but Lenny had to come up with $1200 to get the key.

That was it for the Canyon. It was back to Hollywood Boulevard, poring over the newspaper, checking the bulletin boards at Ralph's and Hughes's markets. They drove up and down streets with long Spanish names like Sierra Bonita and Camino Palmero, where the building supervisors were uniformly rude and unsympathetic to dogs. The Subaru's radiator was shot. Lenny had to put water in every fifteen minutes. In between looking at horrible apartments Lenny and Linda would stop at the Denny's or the Tiny Naylor's or Ben Frank's, greasy spoons which did not charge for refills of coffee and where they could wait for the overworked Subaru to cool down.

Linda wanted Lenny to subscribe to something called *The Homefinders' Guide*, a listing service which cost thirty-five dollars and provided the subscriber with daily listings of rental properties all over town. Linda was drawn by a *Homefinders* ad in the *Herald-Examiner:* "Gst Hse. Hwd Hls., Pets & Kids OK, Use of Htd. Pl., $185." Lenny explained to Linda that these rentals did not exist, they were fictitious draws printed in the paper to get people to lay out that thirty-five-dollar one-time fee. "If the places really did exist," Lenny asked, "how long do you think they'd last? They're rented to somebody's brother as soon as the listing is called in."

Linda knew Lenny was telling the truth, which only made her more depressed. Her back hurt from the night in the Subaru. Even the dog was getting sick. There was thick crust all over Daisy's eyes, and she did not want to play. Linda tried to run the dog in Poinsettia Park that night, but Daisy just wanted to sleep on the yellowed, dry grass. Linda slept for forty-five minutes, Lenny for thirty.

The second day Lenny and Linda looked at five places. All were on either Hollywood Boulevard or Franklin Avenue, between Cahuenga and La Brea. All were similar. They had sparkly sprayed-stucco ceilings, bathrooms with leaky faucets that could barely hold one person, noisy pipes, creaking elevators and filthy, tiny swimming pools that were not in use. Their prospective neighbors, in all cases, were hookers. The real crunch, though, was price. Each of those five pitiful apartments cost at least $500 per month. Lenny could not believe how the prices had gone up since they had last been in Los Angeles.

There was only one thing to do. They could not spend another night in the Subaru. Linda gave Lenny a half Quaalude, watched him take it, and then told him what they both knew they had to do. That morning they had driven by the Hamilton Arms. They had both pretended not to see that the For Rent sign was still up.

"Lenny," Linda told her husband, "it's a studio. How bad can one room be? We don't need a lot of room. I really don't. If I have you, Lenny, you know I can live anywhere."

Lenny could not look Linda in the eye. He knew she was right. The thought of them living in Mel's old building made his stomach turn, but he had no choice. He revved up the Subaru and headed back for Franklin and LaBrea.

The studio was minuscule and had been thoroughly trashed by the previous tenant who, the super told them, had owned a monkey. The landlord was a big corporation that did not care if its tenants owned pets that wrecked the apartments. They were owned purely as a tax loss. Lenny gave the super one hundred dollars for the first week's rent. The apartment rented for $350, but that was only if the entire month's rent was paid in advance. For an extra fifty bucks, the landlord said, Lenny and Linda could pay "as she goes." However, if they fell behind, the super would just tack a "Pay in Three Days or Quit" notice on their door, and that would be that. If they did not pay, Lenny and Linda would be out on the street at the end of the third day. The super assured them that the corporation that owned the building had "an arrangement" with the marshal's office. If they paid the rent, fine. The super did not really care much either way. He was a Vietnamese refugee who had seen real sorrow and could not feel much for people who willfully hurt themselves.

Lenny and Linda were exhausted, but they spent their second afternoon back in Los Angeles carrying boxes from the Subaru to their new apartment and unpacking. They had to park the car in a loading zone in front of the building because a parking space was forty dollars extra per month, which Lenny thought was pure highway robbery. After they had unpacked the car, Lenny went searching for a parking place. He had to park two blocks away. He stopped at Roman's Liquor Store on the way back and bought a Coca-Cola. He shook his head sadly as he looked at his new home. He just could not believe he and Linda were living at the Hamilton Arms. The realization was so painful it made Lenny wince, feel dizzy, then walk as if he carried a heavy load, which he did.

Now Lenny's final-act curtain went up. He had no job, very little money, and essentially no friends. From a reality of making huge amounts of money, becoming a power in Los Angeles, hobnobbing with the young and the rich, Lenny had gone to the Hamilton Arms, the last stop of those who cannot cope with the world *as it is*. Like all people who cannot cope with the world as it is, Lenny began to lead a fantasy life far richer than his prior real life. To the people who tried to be his friend and offered bread, Lenny answered that he was already eating cake. To the friend who offered to get Lenny a real job, Lenny explained that working for someone else was the fool's way out, and that he did not notice Roy Ash working for anyone else. To the friend who sat with Lenny at the Shanghai Winter Garden and offered money for medical help, Lenny said that he was not sick, and that if certain deals worked out as he expected them to, he would soon be endowing a wing at Cedars-Sinai.

Linda now lived in a perpetual fog of self-hatred and anxiety. She had the sense, however, to get out of the apartment each day. She took temporary jobs as a typist and earned the money they lived on at the Lenny and Linda Dream Factory. She was an excellent typist still and worked every day she cared to. When she did not work, she went to the beach by herself and looked at the ocean. She wondered if the point of it all was somewhere in the ocean.

Lenny lay in bed reading the *Wall Street Journal*, the *Institutional Investor*, and *Forbes*. He would occasionally call up about an advertisement for a five-million dollar apartment complex in West Covina or Palm Springs. He would hatch ideas for novel kinds of financing and write out charts and graphs for them. But he never left the apartment. After all, he might run into Mel.

Mel no longer lived in the Hamilton Arms, of course. Lenny thought that Mel was probably dead. No one that bad could live for long, he thought, which was a perfect sign of just how much he had to learn. Although Lenny and Linda were back in the hurricane, the

Hamilton Arms was the eye of the storm. It was quiet there. And even though Mel was no longer a tenant, they could get Quaaludes right in the building from a man named Mark who lived in a one-bedroom down the hall.

Mark was a screenwriter. He sat in his apartment all day, pounding on an old Royal stand-up portable typewriter, working on a script he told Lenny and Linda was called *The Game of Love*, which was going to make Mark rich. He would not let Lenny or Linda read a single word of it, though, because Mark had read Mario Puzo's advice to writers that had been printed in *Time* and had taken the advice to heart. He kept the clipping on his bathroom mirror so he could read it every morning. One of the rules was, "Never show your work in progress to *anyone*, especially relatives and friends." Another rule was, "Do not confuse money with art. If you are feeling financial pressure, go to the movies and forget about it." Mark modified that rule to read: "If you are feeling financial pressure, sell 'ludes and *really* forget about it." Mark was able to make money selling Quaaludes because he did not take them himself.

Linda told me about the day Mark came home, pounded on their door, and told Lenny and Linda that he had sold *The Game of Love* to a major studio for fifty thousand dollars. He invited his friends out to the Hungry Tiger, Mark's treat, for a celebration dinner. Lenny declined. He had "important papers" to go over for an imaginary deal. Linda asked Lenny if he would mind if she went. He said that he would not, and Linda was out the door. She did not look at Lenny's face when she left because she knew she had hurt his feelings. But Mark had no one to celebrate with, Linda had not been out for dinner in weeks, and she knew Lenny would soon get over it. The idea of Linda cheating on Lenny, the man she loved more than life, was completely ridiculous. She would rather throw herself off Mulholland Drive than hurt Lenny. Besides, Linda would give him a 'lude from her secret stash when she got home. That would cheer him up. Linda knew that Lenny was not really mad at her. She suspected that Lenny was jealous over Mark's big movie sale. They had been in Los Angeles for three weeks, and Lenny had yet to get back into business. Things were just a little slow getting off the ground sometimes, Lenny had told her. Especially when one does not leave one's room for days at a time. All the more reason, Linda thought, for her to go out.

Mark did not have a car, although he told Linda he was going to buy one the next day, maybe an Alfa Romeo. In any case, the two friends walked down La Brea to Hollywood Boulevard, past the hookers who hung out in front of Roman's, then crossed the street to the Hungry Tiger. They sat at the oyster bar. Mark was in a great mood. He ordered everything. Linda, at first, was slightly critical of Mark's extravagance; after all, Mark had not been paid for his script yet. Linda knew that things sometimes fell through, especially in Los Angeles. But Mark was so up, so happy, that Linda could not find it in her heart to let him down. Besides, she had not had a decent meal in a long time, except at home. She ate every tourist delicacy the waiter in a red waistcoat brought to their darkened corner of the dining room.

Mark and Linda had shrimp cocktails to start and crab cocktails for dessert. With their after-dinner armagnac, "just for the hell of it," Mark said, the two split a plate of rich baked clams. They were both so full after that, the walk home took twice as long as it did to get there. Mark stopped by the apartment to see Lenny before he went home to dream of his name on the silver screen. He gave Lenny two Quaaludes, free of charge.

Misery loves company, and clichés become clichés because they are true. Lenny and Linda had other friends in the Hamilton Arms. Mark introduced them to Barbara, who lived in the only two-bedroom apartment in the building. Barbara was the self-appointed house mother at the Hamilton Arms. She had flaming red hair, huge breasts, and loved to tell stories about when she had been the top call girl in Las Vegas and had once taken a ride to Mexico in Frank Sinatra's private jet. All of the stories she told took place before she had moved from Vegas to Los Angeles, which is when she started dealing cocaine. That was twenty years ago. Barbara was not at all like Mark: not only did she deal the stuff, she took it, too. A lot of it. When Barbara thought of you as a close friend she confided her deepest secret: twenty years of doing coke every day had created a hole in the cartilage that separated her nostrils. She demonstrated this destruction by sucking water up her left nostril and blowing it back out through her right. Ten years ago, she said, she was at the top of her profession. She had a huge house with a pool in Nichols Canyon and had Chasen's cater dinner parties with rock stars and famous politicians. After the food, a maid would deposit a gram of pure Merck cocaine on tiny sterling-silver salad plates which sat to the left of each guest. She even had the equivalent of a fancy salad fork, only for cocaine: a tiny crystal version of a snow shovel. Barbara had them specially made by Tiffany.

What happened? "I got busted," Barbara told Linda. "Someone, and I know who it was, tipped off the police. They caught me with a couple of pounds of coke and $250,000 in cash. The arrest report said that they had found an ounce and five thousand dollars. Those cops must have gotten pretty fucking high, that's all I have to say."

Like Lenny, Barbara was starting all over again at the Hamilton Arms. The problem was that her old customers, mostly very famous rock stars, had found someone else with cocaine in Nichols Canyon. They did not want to buy their ounces and pounds of coke from someone who was starting over at the Hamilton Arms. Barbara complained and compared the situation to *Catch-22*. The rock stars only wanted to buy their drugs in a pleasant and high-class atmosphere; Barbara could only escape the Hamilton Arms if she did business with her former customers. "It's just not fair," Barbara said. "And would you believe it—I helped out all those guys when they were just starting out, and I don't have a single gold record to hang on my wall." Barbara kept her huge color television on twenty-four hours a day. It was she, the Blanche DuBois of the drug trade, who got Lenny and Linda interested in watching daytime game shows.

Lenny and Linda had only the little black and white Panasonic set, so they preferred to watch television over at Barbara's. The three of them sat quietly on Barbara's couch, drank beers, and watched "Family Feud." Barbara talked nonstop as soon as the show, her favorite, was through. Barbara's stories were white noise for Lenny. Her voice was a constant background hum that somehow took Lenny's mind off the chaotic hell which was his inner life.

They were, however, at least for the moment, well stocked with Quaaludes. Mark *gave* Lenny the rest of his stash the day the contracts for *The Game of Love* came in the mail. A little over one hundred 'ludes. Lenny gave twenty pills to Linda, as a present, and kept the rest for himself. He hid his stash in the back of the Panasonic.

Lenny and Linda stayed up far into the night, blasted into peacefulness by the drug. They slept far into the day. In the few hours of nondrugged wakefulness allotted to them, they schemed and made plans. They watched television with Barbara. Linda stayed away from work for a few days.

Lenny and Linda's five hundred dollars went gradually, the flow slowed by Linda's income. But that income was never large. Linda was not, after all, a robust picture of mental health.

Linda never worked at one place for more than a couple of days. She never got paid much more than minimum wage. Sometimes her temporary employers were stunned with her skill (Linda, on a good IBM, could type close to 120 words per minute) and gave her ten or twenty extra dollars in an envelope, a bonus, on her last afternoon at a particular place. She moved around too quickly to make friends. That was all right with Linda. She did not feel that she deserved friendship. Since she lost the baby, she was always just two or three steps outside of herself, making sure that she stayed somber, stayed regretful, stayed guilty. She was always watchful. She took Quaaludes, but far fewer than Lenny. She often dropped her first 'lude of the day as soon as she got home from work. Lenny was usually still in bed, the trade papers and *Wall Street Journals* spread out on the covers, his eyes glazed over, a stinking pile of half-smoked Viceroys in an overflowing ashtray.

One morning in this period something stirred in Linda. She made Lenny fresh-squeezed orange juice, coffee, toast, eggs scrambled to perfection. It was nine o'clock in the morning. The last time Lenny had been up at nine in the morning had been in Santa Cruz. Linda let him sleep until breakfast was ready. She woke her husband with a kiss, set the tray down on the bed, and opened the windows to let in the pleasant California breeze, which blew even at the Hamilton Arms. Lenny was pleasantly hung over. He was also starving. Lenny and Linda shared the plate of eggs, but Lenny ate everything else. After breakfast, Linda did the dishes. "No game shows today, Lenny," Linda yelled to her husband, who was in the shower. "I've planned a big day for us."

Lenny was still groggy after a hot-and-cold-water shower, but as he got dressed he did notice that the apartment was completely cleaned. Everything was neat and in its place. Linda had been up early and had obviously been working for hours.

"Come on, Lenny, let's go." Linda practically dragged her husband out of the apartment, into the elevator, and down to the Subaru. Linda had had the car washed, too.

"When did you do all this?" Lenny asked.

"Never mind," said Linda. "Get in. I'm driving."

Lenny obeyed. "Where are we going?" he asked.

"That," said Linda, laughing and turning her sparkling eyes on her confused but happy husband, "is for me to know and you to find out. Here," she said and handed him a red bandanna. "Put this over your eyes. You know, like a blindfold."

"No way," said Lenny. "I want to see where we're going."

"Suit yourself," said Linda. She started the car and drove them west, toward the beach. Linda took the long way, straight down Sunset, past the Roxy, past the Beverly Hills Hotel, over the San Diego Freeway, past Brentwood, the Palisades, then the long swoop down and they were at the Coast Highway. It was one of those clear winter days that made the Pacific Ocean sparkle like a huge blue jewel.

"Come on, Linda," Lenny said. "I don't have time for this kind of stuff. I've got some important meetings today."

"No, Lenny," Linda said. She took Lenny's hand in hers. "We have important meetings today. You and me. That's our meeting."

Linda knew that Lenny did not have any important meetings that day, nor had he had any important meetings for a long time. He was in no shape for even one important meeting. She drove up the coast, past Malibu, then turned off at Trancas. She parked the Subaru on a cliff above a particularly deserted stretch of beach.

Linda carried the picnic basket and led the way. She held Lenny's hand, guided him down the winding stairway of rock. Daisy followed close behind. When they hit the beach, Linda reached into the picnic basket and handed Lenny a new pair of Vvarnet sunglasses, the kind that really keep out the sun. Lenny realized that they cost at least seventy dollars. They were exactly the same as a pair he had admired in an *Esquire* ad. Lenny wondered why Linda was being so good to him.

The dark lenses of the sunglasses shielded Lenny's eyes from the bright winter sun. His hangover evaporated. He watched Linda spread a big red blanket out on the sand and anchor the corners with thick paperback novels. Linda took off her shirt and lay down.

"Come on, Lenny," she said. She looked up at Lenny, shielded her face with a raised right hand. Linda squinted. "You could use a little color yourself," she said. "Lie down here with me."

Lenny slowly removed his worn pink oxford-cloth shirt and lay down next to his wife. He looked at her, smiled, and fell asleep.

The weather was spectacular for a day at the beach. The smog burned off completely in the hour that Lenny slept. Linda did not want Lenny to get sunburned. She woke him.

"Let's take a walk, Lenny," Linda suggested.

Lenny looked up and down the beach. He could see no sign of human life. About a hundred yards north, in the sparkling breakwater, two sheepdogs tugged at a blue Frisbee. Their owners were nowhere in sight. Daisy barked at them.

"Let's go that way," Lenny said, pointing. "Maybe we'll find a friend for Daisy."

Lenny and Linda walked quietly, hand in hand. When they reached the dogs, Linda grabbed the loose Frisbee and tossed it in the surf. The dogs went wild, jumping through waves. They both caught the Frisbee at the same time. Neither would let go. The two dogs swam back to the beach, each holding a corner of the blue platter in its mouth. Daisy watched it all and cried for the attention of her beloved Lenny.

"Isn't this great, Lenny?" Linda asked.

Lenny was lost in thought.

"Lenny, doesn't this remind you of Santa Cruz?" Linda said.

"What?"

"This is like Santa Cruz. There's no smog. You can breathe out here. I can't believe we never do this. We just stay in the apartment all the time. I mean, can't you *think* better out here?"

"I think wherever I am," Lenny said sharply. "I'm always thinking, trying to get us somewhere decent."

"I know, Lenny." Linda was silent on the walk back the other way, back toward the picnic basket and lunch.

Lenny sat down on the red blanket as Linda removed many foil-covered packages from the wicker hamper. Lenny was hungry. He grabbed one of the packages and opened it.

"Here, Lenny," Linda said. "Use a plate." Lenny put the fried chicken on the paper plate and started on a drumstick. He was not used to being in the sun. Lenny was sweating. The sweat was making him want a Quaalude. In the rush to leave that morning, Lenny had forgotten to take a pill. A drop of sweat fell off the end of Lenny's nose and mixed with the grease on the white paper plate. He watched the sweat and grease and did not pay attention to what Linda was saying.

"Lenny, aren't you listening to me?"

"I'm sorry," Lenny said.

"Lenny, what are we doing here? What are we doing in Los Angeles? Don't you remember how happy we were in Santa Cruz?"

"That's nothing," Lenny said slowly, "compared to how happy we're going to be in Los Angeles. I know what I'm doing this time. I know what I have to do now. You think I'm a failure and need to run away already?"

"I just thought you would enjoy a day at the beach, Lenny," she said. "That's all."

"It was a good idea. But we've got to be getting back pretty soon. I've got some figures to work up on this new deal. And I'm getting a little bit of a headache from all this sun. Do you have anything?"

Linda knew what Lenny meant by "headache," and she knew what he meant by "anything." "I don't have any pills, Lenny," she said. "What about a beer?"

Lenny took the beer, set down his chicken, and stared out to sea. He drained the beer in two big gulps. The sun was hot, and his head was not getting any better. Linda's purse was on the blanket next to him. It was a bright blue vinyl sack. Lenny had brought it home one day from the sports shop in Santa Cruz. He picked up the purse and emptied its contents on the blanket.

"Lenny," Linda said. "What are you doing?"

"There might be something in here. You might have forgotten you had something. There might be a pill."

Linda reached over for the purse, took it from Lenny's loose grasp. She gathered her wallet, cigarettes, lipstick, and change and put them back in the purse slowly and with care.

"I told you," she said. "There's nothing. I might have one or two at home."

"Is there any more chicken?" Lenny asked.

"Sure," Linda said. She was grateful that Lenny dropped the subject. She handed Lenny a couple of wings and a plastic dish of coleslaw. The two of them ate in silence.

Linda saw Lenny pouring salt on his chicken. She knew that salt was bad for Lenny. She knew that it could, at the least, make his headache worse. In the long run, if Lenny kept it up, the salt could contribute to a heart attack. Then Linda said, "Lenny, please. You shouldn't use that much salt. There's a lot of salt already on it."

Lenny threw his plate of chicken in the sand. He looked up at the blue, cloudless sky. He raised his right hand and cracked Linda across the face with his open palm. It made a sharp smack. "Don't tell me what to do," he said sharply.

Linda covered where Lenny had hit her for the first time with her left hand. She began to cry. Her face hurt, but the look in Lenny's eyes hurt Linda much more. At that moment Linda did not recognize Lenny. He was somebody else. He had been somebody else for a long time.

But now he was Lenny again: a paralyzed, disbelieving Lenny. "Oh, God," he said. "Oh, my God. I'm sorry. Jesus, I'm so sorry."

Linda was silent. She gathered up the picnic basket, the blanket, the garbage of their lunch, and walked up the hill to the Subaru. Lenny followed, stumbling along about ten steps behind. Linda got into the car, waited for Lenny, then started the engine and headed back toward town. She did not take Sunset this time. Linda took the freeway. It was quicker. She wanted to be home and the day to be over.

Lenny did not say a word on the trip back from Trancas. He stared out the window. He kept his hands on his knees, palms down. He pressed down so that his hands would stop shaking. He looked at the rearview mirror on the passenger side of the Subaru, and some part of his mind registered that the glass mirror was cracked. If he had looked at his face in that mirror, Lenny would have seen himself broken into hundreds of pieces.

When they got home, Linda still could not bring herself to look at Lenny. She made herself busy with chores. She put away the picnic hamper, unwrapped a blue-paper package of sheets from the laundry, returned a dish to Barbara down the hall.

Lenny locked himself in the bathroom as soon as they got in. He took the two pills he had hidden at the bottom of a bottle of aspirin and sat on the toilet seat, thinking. When he opened the door, Linda was lying on the bed. He spoke to her then for the first time since hitting her that afternoon.

"Linda," Lenny said, "I swear to you, I swear it's going to be different. I don't know what happened. I swear I will never, ever touch you again. My God, you are the one thing that's good in my life. Linda, I'm getting it together. We don't have to go back to Santa Cruz. I can make it like Santa Cruz *here*."

Linda turned over. She reached out and took Lenny's hand. Her eyes were clear and dry.

"It's all right, Lenny," she said. "I know you didn't mean it."

"I didn't, Linda. I love you. I love you more than I have ever loved anyone in my whole life."

"I love you," Linda said.

Lenny hugged his wife. Then he picked up a copy of the *Wall Street Journal.* He showed Linda an article about a group of New York investors. Really big guys, guys who thought big, like Lenny. The article said that they were interested in setting something up in Los Angeles. They were just looking for the right thing. Lenny told Linda that this was it, this was his chance. Lenny had been doing research. He knew what these guys were into. He had made contact with the key investor. They were all coming out to Los Angeles, a group of four, and Lenny was going to take them out to dinner. Lenny said he had been putting something together that was just right for these guys. Everything was going to be all right, Lenny said. In a couple of weeks they could buy the Hamilton Arms and raze the place, turn it into a park just for them and Daisy.

"It's all right," Linda said, squeezing her husband's hand. Linda was not talking about the deal with the guys from New York. She was saying that she had forgiven Lenny for hitting her. She was saying that she loved him. Linda told me later that at that moment, while Lenny was running down the specifics of the deal that he had set up for the guys from New York, she was trying to remember the last entire day that she had been truly happy with Lenny. She thought that it might have been a day shortly after their arrival in Santa Cruz, but she was not sure.

She also wondered if someday she and Lenny might have another baby. The doctors at Dominican, including Dr. Bernbaum, had told her she was basically ready to get pregnant at any time. But Lenny and Linda were usually far too wasted and far too depressed to make love any longer. Once, the drug had encouraged them to make love as often as three or four times each day. Now they barely spoke, let alone made love.

But Lenny could not hear Linda's thoughts any longer, so now he simply continued talking about how he actually knew about one of the guys who was coming out from New York. The guy had been at a big oil company, maybe Standard of California, and he had super-good contacts with people in Saudi Arabia. He was going to start buying up shopping centers and office buildings as if they were packages of Cracker Jack. Lenny had a way for him to do it and recycle the ownership so that it did not look as if the Arabs were buying up the country, but the Arabs got the rents, anyway.

Truth to tell, Lenny's idea was extremely novel and genuinely smart. It involved the Saudis setting up general partnerships of which the small American investor would then be the limited partners. Since the Saudis were putting up such a large amount of money, the U.S. investors would be at minimal risk and yet could feel that they were getting in on what was then the real-estate boom.

Lenny told me the idea, and although I hate the Saudis, I had to admit that it was a hell of an idea. It would give the impression that the Saudis were sharing their opportunities with Mr. and Mrs. America. Lenny's idea was actually brilliant.

But to get the boys from New York to pay attention, Lenny had to give the right idea about just who he was. That was going to be a problem, but Lenny could solve it.

The big meeting, what Lenny considered as the most important dinner of his life, was a little more than a week away. He would have to make an impression on the big boys, and for that he needed a little extra money. He could not take them to Pioneer Chicken in the Subaru.

Alas, the money that Linda brought home from typing was not enough to rent a flat black Mercedes 450 SEL and was not enough for dinner for six at Ma Maison. Lenny had gotten the meeting on the strength of his old reputation as an up-and-comer, an ambitious and smart young guy. He needed a little front money to cement the deal.

Mark was dealing again. He could wait only so long for the studio to pay him the money for *The Game of Love*, then he had to do something. He was back in the Quaalude business and was glad to have Lenny's help. Mark hated dealing. He would much rather be home, typing, instead of running around Hollywood delivering 'ludes. "I'll split the money with you," Mark offered, "if you can get eight bucks a 'lude and you make the connect with these people. These are the real thing, so eight bucks should be no problem."

Eight dollars was fine, Lenny said. So was ten dollars, as it turned out. If Lenny could middle two extra dollars, that was two dollars more he could use for the guys from New York. Mark certainly did not mind. He got his four dollars.

Lenny made the rounds in that week. Fifty pills here, thirty there; Lenny was disciplined about it. There was a lot riding on his meeting: his entire future, his life with Linda. Lenny took the Subaru at night and went to the Rainbow, Le Dome, Carlos and Charlie's, selling Mark's Quaaludes neatly packaged in plastic bags. It did not take very long, maybe a couple of hours each night. Lenny would finish out the week four or five hundred dollars to the good, if he was careful not to dip into his profits.

And he was careful. He took two 'ludes before he went out, just to steel himself for doing business with Mark's scummy customers. There was one guy who bought ten 'ludes every single night. Lenny met him at the Rainbow bar. The guy's name was Moustapha. He was an Iranian who attended UCLA; whose parents had bought him a Ferrari GTS sports car for his twenty-first birthday; and who received an allowance, Lenny was told, of twenty-five hundred dollars a week. He bought only ten at a time because he did not trust himself with a large quantity. "I am not afraid that I will take them myself," Moustapha said, shooting the cuffs of his Bijan suit. "It is the chicks. I am afraid I will give all of them to a chick. In America," said Moustapha, "I fall in love again every night with someone new." Lenny merely nodded in agreement every night and collected a new one-hundred-dollar bill. Once in a while, after he dealt with Moustapha, Lenny would allow himself just one extra 'lude.

The night before the big meeting, Lenny was sent over for a major drop at Le Dome. The buying party was a young punk with dyed red hair who had ordered two hundred dollars' worth from Mark. Mark told Lenny that when he saw red-dyed hair, he should make a gesture with his left hand, and then the red-dyed-hair gentleman would meet Lenny at the famous circular bar of Le Dome. (The bar had once been the reception area for an advertising agency, but that was when advertising was important and bars were straight.)

Lenny spotted Mr. Red-Dyed Hair immediately at a table with five other boys and girls who looked as if they could be blown away by the slightest breath of bad news. Lenny scratched his nose with his left hand. As he did, he glanced over at the bar.

At the far end of the circle sat Joel. He looked slightly different, but not that different, Lenny thought. His face looked puffy, as if he might be taking large doses of Prednisone. (Lenny was a great expert in all forms of drug reactions, as many drug addicts are.) Joel wore a full Encino ensemble: tight pressed jeans, an open-necked pressed and tailored shirt, a heavy gold chain, Porsche sunglasses, and three gold bracelets. He was not with Rochelle. He was with two teeny boppers in baby-blue spandex tops and jeans. Lenny figured that Joel must have given the bartender a little something to get let in with those two boppers. There were laws about those things. Then Lenny figured that he would take the piece, the little S & W Python that he carried with him on these rounds, and maybe just get himself clear by putting a few rounds right into Joel's skull.

Lenny felt in his jacket pocket for the gun. He suddenly felt so crazed with anger that he had to grasp the side of the bar to support himself against dizziness. An arm touched his shoulder. It was Red-Dyed Hair. He patted Lenny on the back and handed him two hundreds. Lenny reflexively passed over an envelope with twenty 'ludes. He looked at Red-Dyed Hair. Lenny was sure he had seen him interviewed on Phil Donahue, perhaps at the same moment that he had seen Barbara taking water in one nostril and blowing it out the other. Red-Dyed Hair had invented some new way to lose weight or some new kind of music or something that made him rich while Lenny stayed poor.

When Lenny turned around, Joel was gone. Lenny rushed outside, but Joel was not there, either. The spandexed girls were gone, too. Lenny figured that Joel had spotted Lenny and had gotten a little scared. He probably had his car right out in front, anyway. Lenny made a mental note that when his deals went through, he would kill Joel. He did not want to jeopardize the meeting the next day by driving over to Joel's and shooting up his house.

On the way home, though, Lenny did take two more 'ludes than he usually would have. Once he got home, he told Linda what he had seen. Linda told him to forget about it and to think about the meeting instead.

Lenny wanted me to come to the meeting. I know that I have pretty much dropped out of this narrative, but that is because I did not see much of Lenny and Linda for a long time. I visited them twice in Santa Cruz, before the fall. Back then I often talked to Lenny every day of the week on the telephone. But when he fell apart, he kept more to himself. Our paths crossed on a systematic basis only in one way. Lenny was a member of an organization that raised money for lost and abandoned dogs.

I had written several articles about the plight of lost dogs. Now I had become, in a small way, the hero of the lost-dog saviors of Los Angeles. I was constantly invited to address groups of touching men and women whose lives were devoted to those heartbreaking, totally innocent creatures who are found scurrying through streets and alleys, terrified beyond endurance by any noise or sudden movement, their whole world shattered by having been abandoned. The looks of utter terror on their faces are enough to make me write a column asking for capital punishment for anyone who abandons a dog and mean it.

Lenny felt the same way. Like the good friend he was, he read all my columns. Like the animal lover he was, he gave fifty or a hundred dollars from his dealing to animals each month, even when he literally could not afford to put gasoline into the Subaru. The little old people in the organization were entranced by Lenny's fast talking and forceful advocacy for animals. Lenny once cleaned himself up, dragged himself out of the Hamilton Arms, and brought himself to a meeting of the county supervisors on an ordinance protecting lost dogs from so-called "medical" experiments. Of all the speakers, only Lenny brought the crowd to its feet when he broke down in the middle of his speech and started to cry as he talked about torturing the only perfectly good friend that man has.

Lenny and I stayed in touch through the organization and also through his plans and schemes. He had always believed that I was secretly rich and could understand any intricacy of finance. Whenever he thought of a new wrinkle, he called me to ask me my opinion. The laugh was that he usually interrupted me while I was writing a script about putting people in chicken suits to ask about the tax treatment of closely held corporations. Still, I had gone to law school and I did know a little something about his subjects. We would talk for an hour or more about all the details of one of Lenny's scams, and then Lenny would thank me profusely and resume thinking. He claimed that the 'ludes allowed him to think far more clearly about major financial deals than if his brain were cluttered up with details such as an undrugged person would have to think about. As if Lenny's brain were not a swarming wasp's nest of self-hatred and rage. As if Lenny could follow up on any of his ideas beyond a telephone call to me, and, as it happened, a fateful meeting.

As I said, Lenny wanted me to come to dinner with the guys from New York, the major hitters, Billy Saperstein and Michael Fuchs. The Saudis had cleverly gotten Jews to manage their money, purely as a public-relations gesture. I had written a novel about a financial catastrophe that had been widely read in New York (so the publisher claimed), and Lenny thought the heavy hitters would probably know who I was. "Anyway, they sure as hell will know who your father is."

The day of the big dinner, Billy Saperstein called Lenny. Lenny had made Linda stay home that day just so that she could answer the telephone and say, "Capital Preservation Equities, good morning," for obvious reasons. Lenny told Billy Saperstein that Lenny would pick them up at the Beverly Wilshire Hotel at eight o'clock and take them to Ma Maison. "The best chef there has left to start his own place, but it's still a cute place to go for a simple French dinner."

Billy Saperstein said that Ma Maison was just fine with him.

Lenny went out and rented a Mercedes 450 SEL, flat black, just as he had wanted, from Budget Rent-A-Car on La Cienega (yes, in Los Angeles, Budget rents the most expensive cars). He picked up the suit he had bought at Carroll and Company for the dinner. He had talked them into opening a house account by dropping the right names with the right tone of indignation. He went to Bullock's-Wilshire and bought Linda a navy blue dress that was from the designer floor but had been reduced to $185. He also stopped at Ma Maison at lunch and gave the captain, a vain man with a drug habit, ten 'ludes to be sure to get the very best table in the place, right next to where Swifty Lazar usually sat with the beautiful Mary. The captain nodded and pocketed the pills.

I was to meet Lenny there. He did not want the SEL to be too crowded. Plus, it would make the right kind of impression that I had a Benz, too, as if Lenny traveled in the crowd where everyone had a Benz.

Making a good impression meant a lot, whether you were investing money for the Saudis or selling dope to bass guitarists. Lenny had learned that. He and Barbara had lengthy skull sessions before the big night, planning every detail of how to make the right impression. Barbara told him that he should definitely get himself some tasseled loafers from Brooks Brothers downtown, even if he did get headaches from the smog down there. She also told him that he should buy Linda a single strand of pearls to go with her blue dress from Bullock's-Wilshire. It is a measure of Lenny's condition that he, a graduate of NYU—more important, a former salesman at Bloomingdale's—had to be told about these things by Barbara, a former hooker from Clark County, Nevada.

At about five in the afternoon, Lenny went out to the Sunset Car Wash to get the Benz washed and porcelainized. He wanted it to look as if a chauffeur cared for it. By the time he got home, he was beginning to feel worried. After all, it was entirely possible that there had been developments, major changes, in tax laws relating to limited partnerships that would make it literally impossible for Lenny to put together his idea. Billy Saperstein and Mike Fuchs might laugh at him. They might say, "Hey, Lenny, the IRS made all that kind of stuff illegal a few years ago." Lenny frantically called me to make me swear that I did not know of anything that would keep the deal from happening as far as new IRS regs were concerned.

"I'm not an expert in that," I told him. "I don't even practice law anymore."

"I know," he said, "but as far as you know, they can't think I'm a total schmuck just for suggesting it, can they? I mean, it's not as if I'm writing my name on the wall in shit, is it?"

"Lenny," I said, "it's a fantastic idea. It really is. If I were those guys, I would buy it right at the dinner table. It's brilliant." I said it and I meant it.

Still, Lenny was a little nervous as he was getting dressed. He was ready a good fifteen minutes before Linda. He glared at her as she dressed in their tiny bathroom which still smelled of monkey, as if she might be trying to sabotage him by being late. "I'm just trying to look pretty for you," she said. "That's all. I can't get ready as fast as a man can."

And, in fact, she did look wonderful that night. From some mystic reserve, she drew the strength to look like the beautiful, chic, utterly confident wife of a Pound Ridge stockbroker. She literally glowed when she walked into the restaurant, Daisy Buchanan with the man who would shame the Great Gatsby.

Before Lenny and Linda left the apartment, the Vietnamese superintendent came by. In an utterly monotonic voice, he reminded Lenny that he was a few days late in the rent. "It's pay up or get out," he said. "I don't make the rules."

Lenny started to tell him that if the dinner went well that night, he would soon own the whole square mile surrounding the Hamilton Arms. But the superintendent, whose name was Ng, walked away, leaving Lenny to tell himself about his future.

Mark came by to wish Lenny luck. Mark told Lenny that he, Mark, had been almost totally down and out before he sold *The Game of Love* and that Lenny could count on one thing, which was that the darkest hour is just before dawn. He hugged Lenny, shook Lenny's hand, and pressed five 'ludes into Lenny's palm. "When I sold my script," he said, "I dropped two 'ludes before the meeting, even though I never take them. It was just to show how relaxed I was. It didn't matter what I *said* to those guys. They knew I was totally confident and totally relaxed, so it all worked out great. Image, man, that's everything."

Lenny did not need any further persuasion. While Linda applied her eyeliner, Lenny crushed up a 'lude, mixed it with soda water and orange juice, added another half just to be sure, and then swallowed the concoction. He felt a lot better before he put down the glass on the Formica counter. This was going to be the night that proved that Lenny might have been down but was never out. Lenny could already see himself explaining to the interviewer for *Forbes* how the whole business plan with the Saudis had come to him. He was thinking about whether he could get me to use my connections (by then, nonexistent) with the *Wall Street Journal*, to get a front-page story about his rise from the ashes in real estate.

When he and Linda walked out to their gleaming 450 SEL, it was as if God had told them that they might now have not only a second, but a third chance. Lenny in his tan gabardine suit, Linda in medium blue from Bullock's-Wilshire, the car, Daisy looking at them through the window, Barbara standing at the curb to wish them well, the entire scene looked like the beginning of the comeback trail for Lenny and Linda Brown.

Lenny could feel that something great was about to happen. He felt happy and confident as he threaded his way through traffic on Sunset Boulevard. When they turned off Sunset onto Crescent for the descent through Beverly Hills to the hotel, Lenny picked up Linda's hand and squeezed it in the same dear old way. *I love you.* Linda squeezed back, *How much? A lot,* Lenny squeezed back.

When they pulled up into the all-Chinese-staffed parking lot at the Beverly Wilshire, Lenny spotted two well-dressed, confident young men whom he knew to be the honchos. Before he leaped out, he turned to Linda and stroked her cheek. "No matter how big I get after tonight," he said, "no matter what happens, I want you to know something. Nothing in my life has ever been worth one hair on your head. If God ever made an angel, it was you." Then he kissed her on the cheek and got out to meet the heavy-hitters. That was the last time Linda ever heard a loving word from Lenny.

ɦARA-KIRI

It was always the same. When Lenny was by himself or with Linda, he did just fine. He stayed out of trouble even if he did take Quaaludes. He could assert some modest balance in his life, some gyroscopic, autonomous inertia that kept him going without wild highs or lows. But when other people came into his life, he was in trouble. He never got into that kind of trouble with me, because he and I made a conscious decision that we would not compete from the earliest stages of our relationship. I would be the artistic one, and he would be the business star. But when Lenny got around men he saw as competition, especially men he saw as besting him in the competition for the good things of life, he lost control. That had been his story with Joel, with the customers at Bloomingdale's, with Billy Saperstein.

Lenny did not remember what should have been immediately memorable as soon as he read about Billy Saperstein in the *Wall Street Journal.* He knew Billy Saperstein. In fact, in 1969 he and Billy Saperstein had been in the same class at NYU about the Chief Modern Poets of England and America. Lenny had hated Billy Saperstein then. "Sap," as he liked to be called, was the only son of a family that was the largest private-label manufacturer of children's underwear in the world. Sap had a Porsche when he was still in school. Sap openly made fun of Lenny when he ran into Lenny working at

Bloomingdale's. And now Sap was in charge of investing about three billion dollars of Saudi money, which was not much to King Khalid but was sure a lot to Lenny. And there Sap stood on the stairs of the Beverly Wilshire in a Paul Stuart suit, looking as if he owned the fucking place when he was really just staying there, the same as any other guest. The other fellow looked like a little MBA wimp Sap had taken with him to carry around his putz, as Lenny told me later.

Sap had not been taking Quaaludes steadily for over a year, so Sap immediately, from the first telephone call, had known that Lenny was the same Lenny he had known at NYU. Truth to tell, Sap had always thought that Lenny was an extremely imaginative kind of guy, a total hustler, and Sap had been a few beats behind in the news he had gotten from the coast. He thought that Lenny was still coining money. Sap frankly knew that Lenny probably did have a great idea, and Sap figured that he could probably get it away for peanuts.

Lenny bounded out of the car and strode up to Sap. "Hey, buddy," Lenny said. "Long time no see. I guess there's been a few changes since Washington Square, huh?"

Billy Saperstein said that he always knew Lenny was going places, that Lenny still had the prettiest wife in the world, and that Lenny and Sap were about to become so rich that they would rebuy the Loeb Center and rename it the "Hustler Center."

As the foursome drove to Ma Maison, Sap and Lenny kept up a running banter about people they had known from college. Sap also paid repeated, lavish, only slightly mocking compliments to Lenny and Linda on how well they were doing out in this crazy place, "where they don't even have trees that have leaves that have points."

Sap allowed that he and his wife, Trish, had just bought a country place up near Lakeville, Connecticut, and as far as he was concerned, if the Saudi deals worked, he was just going to go up there and stay there pretty much forever.

Linda thought that the conversation was going well. As far as she could tell, there was every likelihood that over crepes stuffed with salmon, Lenny could carry off a major coup in real estate. There was already a little talk about the subject of where to put all the Saudi money by the time they got to the restaurant. As far as Linda could see, things were moving along beautifully.

The problems began when they got into the foyer of Ma Maison. The captain to whom Lenny had given ten 'ludes must have taken all ten of them, because he was nowhere in sight. Lenny and Linda did have a reservation, but the barely civil personage who runs Ma Maison, just for the heck of it, told Lenny that the only place they could put him was against the far wall, where the tourists sit.

Lenny's blood froze with fear and anger. Sap had probably been to Ma Maison before. He undoubtedly knew which were the good tables. He would undoubtedly know just what the score was with Lenny if Lenny could not get a better table. Lenny spoke in a low voice to the owner, but the owner answered in a loud voice that the table by the wall was the only table they had.

As they were being conducted to the table, Lenny told Sap that the owner was just doing this as a trick, as a joke because he knew Lenny so well. Sap believed Lenny, as far as Linda could tell, but by then Lenny was so jacked up that he went to the tiny men's room, crushed four 'ludes with the back of his watch, then swallowed the powder with a chaser of water from the tap. It was essential that he be cool.

Lenny also knew that businessmen in New York considered it important to drink whiskey. So he ordered a martini for himself and one for Linda. By the time the drinks arrived, Lenny was really going from the four 'ludes he had virtually inhaled. A serious conversation had already started about the possibilities of a *nationwide* limited partnership in which the Saudis seemed to be giving the ordinary American a chance to get into the commercial real-estate business right alongside the richest people in the world. Linda recalls that Sap actually told Lenny that the concept was "brilliant" and wanted to know if Lenny had told anyone else. The other guy, Michael Fuchs, kept muttering about the tax consequences to the Saudis, but Lenny insisted that if you got enough tax lawyers in a room, typing on an infinite number of typewriters, reading an infinite number of tax treatises, you would certainly, unquestionably, come up with the right answer. Sap agreed. Sap had to admit that Lenny was a savvy guy. The project had just the right public-relations touch. It had just the right capital-gains angle for the Saudis. It looked like the kind of thing that would let Americans know that the Saudis were their pals and make a lot of money, too.

Lenny started to feel pretty damned good. He downed his martini in two gulps, then ordered another. He sneaked a 'lude with his second drink. In a moment he was flying. He was flying so high that when Michael Fuchs started to ask if the limited partnership would have to be blue-skyed in all fifty states, Lenny just stared at him and said, "I don't worry about details. I think about the big parts." He made a sweeping gesture which knocked the bread bowl onto the floor just as the owner was walking by with Susan Anton. Sap looked a little embarrassed, so Linda quickly began talking about how wonderful life must be in Lakeville, Connecticut. That distracted Sap, but Michael Fuchs kept staring at Lenny as if he knew that something funny were going on.

When the hors d'oeuvres came, Lenny was having trouble forming words of more than two syllables. He tried to answer questions about stepped-up depreciable basis, but his words were slurred. In fact, by that time, he had only a vague idea of what the conversation was about.

Michael Fuchs, a weasely little guy with the light blue eyes that invariably belong to troublemakers, sensed a chink in Lenny's armor. He began to ask Lenny whether Lenny contemplated that this would be a section 355 transaction under the code. He picked at his salmon mousse as he asked, to give the impression that the answer was extremely important.

"I don't worry about that shit," Lenny said irritably. "Don't you have any lawyers left in New York?"

"Of course," Michael Fuchs said. "We have a full staff at our office, and we have retained Cravath, Swaine & Moore as our counsel. I think that some idea of the tax consequences down the road would be helpful. It might show our principals that your plan is carefully thought out."

I could see that Lenny was getting ready to tell Michael Fuchs to fuck himself. I had stayed quiet all through the meal, but this was really intolerable. "You know," I said, "you're asking Lenny questions that wouldn't even come up in a lawyer's office until the fifth or sixth meeting. Plus, you're asking them before anybody, including you, even knows whether it would be better for this to be a three fifty-one transaction or a three fifty-five transaction. Why are you doing this? We know you're a smart guy."

Michael Fuchs looked abashed and then played with his salmon mousse again. He looked at me and smiled. "We wouldn't be concerned if we were listening to your plan, Ben," he said. "But we feel as if we might be staking a lot of money and our reputation on Lenny's plan, and everyone knows that Lenny's a smart guy, too, but he's had a few problems."

Before I could even speak, Lenny looked up and stared at Michael Fuchs. I thought he might hit Michael Fuchs and make blood come out of Michael Fuchs's little nose onto his striped Paul Stuart shirt. But Lenny did not do that. Instead, he summoned a calm look, a gentle voice (although Linda and I could detect the strain), and said, "I think you would be making a major mistake to blame me for a tentative ruling by the IRS that closed down almost every real-estate tax-shelter specialist in California for a year. But if you want to, you can. I can always take this plan to Genstar."

Sap said, "Hell, no, Lenny. We love the idea. It's just that we talked to a few people we ran into at the hotel about you, and they said you have been into some pretty serious stuff." He cleaned his tortoiseshell glasses with his Chipp tie and said, "I still think you've got a great idea. It's just that if we take back the idea, we want everybody in New York to know that you're a really buttoned-down guy who's thought everything out just right, so that if someone comes in and starts telling stories about you, we've got the proof that they're full of shit."

"Well, that's fair," Lenny said. "If you write down your questions, I'll give you a letter answering all of them within a week." Lenny sounded like a guest on "Meet the Press."

"We aren't Cravath, Swaine & Moore," I said, "but I have a lot of friends who know tax, and we can at least give you a basis for knowing that Lenny has done a lot of really thorough work on the concept." I felt it was important to say "we," and I wish I had said it earlier and more often.

"That's all we ask," Sap said.

"I'll get you a letter in a few days," Michael Fuchs said. "But it will be a pretty tough letter. You'd better be prepared for some serious homework."

The main course came and we ate in a cheerful mood. We talked about why television was so terrible, about how silly life in Los

Angeles was, about the thousand different ills that flesh is heir to. All of us talked, that is, except Lenny, who ate his food silently, ordered another martini, and, to those of us who knew him, was getting so 'luded out that he hardly could tell where he was. At least that's what we thought until the check came and Michael Fuchs reached for it.

Lenny whipped out his hand and grabbed the check. "No," he said, "let me. Then you can tell the fuckers who said all that bad stuff about me that at least I can still buy a decent meal. You can tell the fucking Arabs that you weren't being taken out by a total derelict."

Michael Fuchs withdrew his hand and glanced meaningfully at Billy Saperstein. Sap looked sadly at Lenny.

"I mean, I don't want you to go back to your Arab friends who wipe their asses with their bare hands and have them think you were out to dinner with a guy who didn't have a Harvard MBA and who hadn't inherited a children's ready-to-wear business. It's no sweat for me. I can get plenty of other people to bite on this idea," Lenny said.

"Listen," Sap said, "you're making a mistake. We really like your idea. We really think it's got a lot of potential. I think you should come to New York and pitch it to the real bosses, if you know what I mean." Sap smiled ingratiatingly as he spoke, and I wondered why Lenny was so angry at him.

By now we were all starting to get up. Lenny had signed the check, which was a privilege he no longer had, but then the waiters at Ma Maison were far too concerned with Susan Anton than with whether or not Lenny still had a charge at the restaurant. Lenny brushed against Freddy de Cordova's table and knocked a glass of white wine into Janet de Cordova (the perfect party person, according to Joan Didion), which then fell over onto her lap. Lenny did not look. He also knocked against a waiter carrying a plate of strawberries. They, too, went sailing to the ground. Lenny was now the bull in the china shop. Linda started to grasp his arm and say, "Lenny's not feeling well . . ." but Lenny shook her off and said, "Oh, no, if they think I'm a junkie, I'll be a junkie for them."

Sap started to speak, but Lenny cut him off in a loud voice. "I'm sorry I'm not good enough to introduce my pitiful ideas to their fucking stinking Arab friends, but maybe I can be their junkie driver and drive them home to their hotel where their friends can tell them more lies about me."

"I think maybe we should take a cab," Michael Fuchs said.

Lenny wrapped his arm around Michael Fuchs and leered menacingly. "This ain't New York," he said. "I'll take you. You'd have to wait an hour for a taxi. I'm not going to hurt you. I'm your servant. I have to be nice to people like you."

"He's not feeling well," Linda said. "Maybe you should take a cab."

In a seething voice, Lenny spoke just as the valet pulled up in the SEL, still shining, still gleaming brilliantly under the streetlights: "Linda, everybody, get in. I have to take you home."

Amazingly, Linda and the honchos got in. As they started to drive off, I said to Sap, "He's upset now because he worked so hard on his plan, and your friend belittled him. . . ." But Sap was not listening. He was too frightened to listen. He sat in the back seat like the prisoner of a crazed zombie killer, which perhaps he was. For neither the first nor the last time, I was completely powerless to keep something terrible from happening.

I later learned that on the drive home, Lenny gave Michael Fuchs unshirted hell for his attitude. "You have never in your whole life come up with an idea with one-tenth the imagination of my idea for your Arab friends. If you had, you'd be working at Morgan, Stanley, instead of carrying around your little smirk for a bunch of Arabs. When this idea puts the company that did it on the cover of *Fortune*, I hope you'll spend even one minute not looking up your asshole."

No one else talked on the way home. Three blocks before the Beverly Wilshire, on Wilshire Boulevard, Lenny sideswiped a parked car in front of a delicatessen. Lenny did not even slow down. No one in the car said anything. When the car was one block from the hotel, which is to say when Lenny's guests could see where they were, they looked at each other and leaped from the car. They ran across five lanes of traffic, tore up the sidewalk, and ran into the hotel. And that was the end of Lenny's fantasy of greatness in real estate for the count.

Lenny and Linda did not talk much on the way home. Linda stared out the window and watched the world go by. I believe that she had the same kinds of thoughts that Lenny had had that first night over a year before when his world had collapsed and he realized that there was an entire universe of people out there going about their daily routines of buying groceries, caring for a sick relative, taking the bus to work, doing anything that would not make them sick with anxiety and self-loathing and fear. All of those people were traveling effortlessly along life's highway, and Linda was pulling a sledge of scrap metal that weighed ten tons.

I am not going to drag out the rest. When Lenny and Linda got home, Lenny started to take three more 'ludes out of his stash in the back of the trusty Panasonic even as Linda brought Daisy in from her walk. Linda walked over and slapped the pills out of Lenny's hand. "This is it," she said. "We've had enough of your wallowing around and tormenting yourself and everybody else. You're going to stop taking that shit right this minute. You had those people eating out of your hand. You could have been on your way to New York to be handling something really big, and you threw it into a rathole because you were so fucked up on 'ludes that you didn't know what was happening. You didn't know enough not to just cut your guts open and bleed to death in front of everyone. I'm going to work full-time, and you're going into some kind of drug-rehabilitation program. That's the way it's gonna be," she said. "Even if you have to go into the hospital. I love you, Lenny, and I'm not going to let you kill yourself in front of my eyes one minute longer."

Lenny stared at Linda in disbelief. He sputtered in slurred tones about how Michael Fuchs had started it, but he gave up after a moment. It was too lengthy a story for a man on 'ludes and martinis. He bent over and started to pick the pills up off the floor. Linda swatted them out of his hand again. "No," she said. "That's it. It's over," she added. "You're getting straight right now. Right this minute."

"You bitch," Lenny said. "After all I've done for you. After all you've done to me. After you ruined everything in Santa Cruz, now you're turning against me, too. I had to fight with those people all by myself. I've always had to do everything all by myself. Nobody's ever helped me as much as I would help a lost dog I didn't even know. And you dare to tell me I can't take something so that it doesn't hurt so much?" He grabbed Linda by the wrists and threw her backward against the wall. Daisy started to cry. Linda propelled herself forward and threw out her arms to swat the pills out of his hand yet again. He grimaced in anguish, then stepped forward and literally hit her as hard as he could, right across the face, sending her spinning around and then knocking her against the pathetic dining-room table, against which she hit the side of her head. She slumped to the floor, put her hand to her temple, felt blood, and just looked at Lenny through painful and teary eyes.

Lenny could not believe what had happened. He fell to the floor next to her and started to hug her and plead with her to forgive him. She was in too much pain and too stunned to answer. Barbara came to the door, let herself in with the passkey she had, called the paramedics and the police.

An ambulance came and took Linda away to Hollywood Presbyterian, which is to the Dominican Hospital in Santa Cruz what the South Bronx is to Croton-on-Hudson. Two policemen, a Mexican and a huero, came over to tell Lenny that they usually allowed one warning in a wife-abuse case, but that if Linda turned out to be really hurt, he could count on being pulled in to do some heavy time. "And being fucked up on 'ludes ain't gonna get you any points with the judge, man," the Mexican said. He knew the signs right away.

Lenny asked Barbara to drive him to the hospital. She told him to fuck himself. So did Mark. He called me, told me about what had happened. I came over and sat with him. He lay curled up on the bed, smoking one Viceroy after another, rocking back and forth in misery. As I now recall, he did not say anything for almost three hours. I read Mansfield Park but could not really concentrate. At about six in the morning, Lenny went over to the hospital in my car, with me driving. There was a hospital guard outside Linda's room. He was big and black and looked as if he would just as soon hit Lenny as talk to him.

"You her husband?" he asked.

Lenny nodded.

"Then get the hell out of here, boy," he said. "She don't want to see you."

Lenny could not believe it, but the guard told Lenny that Linda was under police protection and that if he didn't get the hell out of there *real* fast, he could just forget about everything except getting his ass in jail. The guard played with his club as he spoke to Lenny.

It was true. A young doctor, whom I will call Tom Morgenstern, had patched up Linda, taken cranial X-rays and a blood screen. He had determined that she had a slight concussion and a small subdermal hematoma in her scalp which would cause no trouble if she lay quietly for a few days. Tom was a smart internist, so he guessed right away who had done the beating. Linda was wired out of her mind with fright and confusion. Her whole center of life had just collapsed into a million shards right in front of her eyes. Her protector, her beloved, had become her tormentor, a threat to her very life. Most painful of all, she saw that she could not do a single thing for him. Not one thing except to make him even crazier than he already was.

Tom talked to her through the night. He told her that she was quite a cut above what they usually saw at Hollywood Presbyterian, but he would give her the same advice he gave the Gutierrez and Washington abused wives. "Get out," he said. "Just get the hell out. You're not doing him any good, and you're not doing yourself any good. Just get out and let life go on without you getting beat up."

Linda might have said that he needed her, but that would have been a long time before. She was just so scared and so confused, and it had been such a long, long time since anything had felt right. She could hardly remember the last time she had been able to get through a day without fear or premonitions of disaster. When Dr. Tom Morgenstern suggested that he get a guard to keep her husband out, she did not argue. She felt so utterly defeated that she hardly knew what to do any longer. That person who had been a beautiful housewife at Ma Maison only a few hours before was as foreign to her as the innocent, enthusiastic girl who had come out from New York two and a half years before. She did not even know who she was anymore. But she liked being in the cool white hospital room, with Tom talking to her in a soothing voice. She just might have a chance at getting some shelter if she could only keep from having to confront Lenny. If she could stay in the room, listen to the air conditioning for a few days, even with the cries from the hall, if she could hear a man like Tom, whose voice was not filled with chaos and fear, whose hands were strong and firm, she might have a little bit of shelter.

Linda gave the OK to have a guard keep Lenny out. She could hear him arguing with the guard, and then she could hear him walk away. Dr. Tom was with her. He told her it would be all right. Dr. Tom had a kindly face with a lot of wrinkles, even though he was only thirty-one. He also had deep brown eyes. He had also been very heavily into 'ludes himself and had an idea of what the best thing to do for addicts was if you were married to one: "Stay the hell away."

At that moment, in her mind, Linda told herself that maybe she would get back with Lenny in a few days, when he had had time to cool off. Then maybe he could start getting himself together. But at some level, she also knew she would never live with Lenny again for the rest of her life.

Lenny and I went home to my house on Mulholland Drive. He watched the sun rise over the San Gabriel Mountains. He sat in a leather rocking chair my parents had once given to me. He drank the coffee that my wonderful wife made for him. He chain-smoked Viceroys and patted my dog's head. My wife and I did not try to talk to him. He simply rocked back and forth in the chair, hugging himself, his cheeks red and shiny, and would not look at either me or my wife. He moaned occasionally, like a wounded, terrified animal. He told Mary, the dog, that he had done something terrible and had lost the only good thing in his life. He soon had made a mark on the floor from where he had moved the chair from his moaning and rocking back and forth. He reminded me of Orthodox Jews beating their breasts begging for forgiveness of their sins on Yom Kippur, or else of a wolf whose mate has been captured. He would not eat any food. At about noon, he asked me to take him to his apartment so that he could take care of Daisy.

As I let him off, he said he just wanted to be alone for a while. "Never," he said, "I never thought it could happen. Everything else, but not this, and I did it to myself." He did not say it in a way which was supposed to be dramatic or even self-pitying. Lenny's tone was of pure, irreplaceable loss.

Because I am not a stone, I went inside Lenny's apartment with him. I watched as he picked up and kissed the dog, who was still with him, and turned on the faithful Panasonic, which had always worked, even after it had been put in the closet for a year. Lenny took the dog out, then came in, took three Quaaludes from the back of the Panasonic and chewed them dry, as if they were Tums. He swallowed a Diet Pepsi with them and then sat in a pitifully ragged easy chair that had once been Linda's favorite seat.

Daisy jumped up and settled onto his lap in one easy, sinuous motion. On the television, a much younger Steve McQueen played a sheriff who carried around a sawed-off rifle. The picture was in black and white. That day everything was in black and white.

"When I was a little boy," Lenny said, "I used to go with my mother when she went shopping at the Hempstead Mall. I would just take a book—the only one I can remember is *The Count of Monte Cristo*—and I would sit on a step and wait for my mother to come out of Saks. I can't remember any other time I had any peace. I remember that when it got really hot, my father would sit out on a fire escape and listen to a baseball game on the radio, with the mosquitoes buzzing all around him. Then he would walk right by me as he went in to go to sleep. I would be there on the couch reading something, and he would just go walking right by me without saying anything.

"Do you know," he said, "that I cannot remember my father ever saying anything at all to me until I was about fourteen years old? Then he was mad at me because I spent my whole allowance on a transistor radio. He thought I should have learned how to make it myself. A transistor radio. He certainly had no idea of how to make them," Lenny added with a laugh.

"My parents used to have a dog. It was a short-haired terrier. They would hit it if it ever tried to get up on the furniture. I was the only person in the house who would let her get up on the furniture. She would sleep with me on my bed until my parents found out, and then they gave her away. Her name was Betsy. I think they gave her away. They might have just had her put to sleep. They were afraid that she would put a rip into the plastic slipcovers they had over the furniture in the living room. God help me, it's true," he said, looking at without seeing Steve McQueen, who was still alive then.

"I remember that every time I got a report card, my mother would read it, and she would ask me what the other kids on the block got. If even one of them had gotten better, she would scream at me for hours about how lazy I was, how embarrassing it was to have a son who just wasted his time reading books while the other kids were getting ahead, getting the kinds of grades that would get them scholarships and get them ahead. She kept it up all through dinner, and my father wouldn't say a word," Lenny said.

"And then I got Linda, by some miracle that I still don't understand. I got Linda, and she never asked me for a thing. Never. You know that? I had to force her to ask for that dance studio. I had to force her to accept that Jaguar. She didn't want them. She wanted to stay home and talk to me and go to dance class, and she never, not once, complained that she had to work. She never talked about the things she had to have if we got rich. She never thought it would last. She just thought we were lucky to have each other. She thought that maybe if we ever got really rich, then maybe, just maybe, we could get a decorator to do our living room. That was all she wanted."

"She wanted for you to have some peace of mind," I said.

"Yes, indeed," Lenny said. "She wanted that and I wanted that, and I never even got close. Not even close. Not even in the best days with Max." He kissed Daisy on the head, and Daisy kissed him back on the lips. He did not stop her. "Linda always hoped that someday we would just go back to New York. That was what she really, really wanted. She wanted to get out of all this shit. She said it was killing me after that deal went down in the *Wall Street Journal*. She said she would work two jobs as a typist if we would just go back to New York. But I kept thinking that I had been close, really close to getting enough money so that I would have some peace of mind. I thought that Joel would put me into some kind of deal or Max would have a comeback or something that would be really big would put me back with the Rolls convertible, and then everything would be all right."

Since I am paid to be a writer, I kept thinking about the boats borne back ceaselessly against the tide, about running ever faster, never getting where we wanted to be, trying vainly to go backward in time to a place where there was peace of mind. Lenny Brown, I thought, is not really so rare. He is only an American, one of many, all thinking that they can achieve the impossible by running a little faster, making a little more money, getting a slightly better table at La Scala. Then they would find Nirvana in some long, impossible dream in the past. Lenny Brown, that perfect American, thought that by work and struggle, he could find something that even the most brilliant philosophers and sages find only by letting go.

"All the time I was working, selling those tax-shelter things, all that time I was running and running and huffing and puffing and busting my balls, and the whole fucking time there were all these guys who were making more money, who could just sit on the toilet all day and their interest would be more than I would make in a year," Lenny said, and then he came to the part I would like to write in skywriting above Los Angeles.

"It didn't bother me back east that I saw other people who had more of everything than I did. Or maybe it bothered me, but not that much, because I just thought, well, that's the way it's meant to be. Maybe I'll get a little something, but the way it's basically supposed to be is the way it is. But when I got to Los Angeles, it was all different. Then, for the first time, it seemed to me as if I could have it all. It seemed to me for the first time that I could have everything and be just as big as I had ever dreamed about being. The most crazy things I had ever dreamed about were happening to guys stupider than I was every goddam day. So I thought, well, schmuck, now's the time and here's the place. *It's all possible here,* so think big. I used to talk about thinking big, but I never meant it. So I start to think really big, and then somebody pulls out the rug. I try and try, and somebody pulls out the rug. And all the time, I think of all those people with their houses in Bel-Air, and they're all laughing and saying, 'Look, putz, we did it. What the hell's wrong with you?' "

Lenny got up and drank a full can of Diet-Pepsi in a few seconds. It has no calories, no nutrients, and so it is easy to swig down. He offered me one, but I have always preferred sodas with sugar, and so he went on.

"This place," he said, "this fucking place, this stinking place," he said, gesturing toward the city. "It was like someone had told me that all the craziness I had kept inside me could come out, and then when it came out someone said, 'Ha ha, the joke's on you. Everyone else can have all those good things, but you can't.' Back east, I never would have expected to have them. Five years ago, I wouldn't even have thought about tables at Ma Maison. Tonight I might have lost my wife because I got so crazy because I didn't get the right one.

"What the hell does it mean when you get so crazy about things that don't mean anything?" he asked.

"I don't know," I said.

"It means you've gotten so crazy that you think you should be able to control the day or the week or how hot it will be that night. It means you think you run everything. It means everything that happens each minute can hurt you. It means you're a cat with whiskers ten feet long." He paused. "It means you hurt all the time." He playfully shook a 'lude out on the palm of his hand and threw it up in the air and caught it in his mouth. He swallowed it dry and then chased it with yet another Diet Pepsi.

"You get so crazy with longing for whatever comes along that you start to do bad things to the only person in the world who really cares whether you live or die. That's what happens. And then you lose her because you're so fucked up trying to stop hurting all the time. And then you might just as well be dead, because then you're never going to catch up."

I had never seen Lenny strip himself so naked. As far as I can recall, I have never heard anyone ever speak so honestly about anything even remotely connected with himself. When I thought that a man of this much sensitivity had been so tortured by anyone, a person or a city, it made me want a Quaalude, too. Lenny, that businessman, so much more sensitive than any paid artist on earth, was in pain.

Lenny and I sat silently for well over an hour. We could hear the traffic on La Brea and the other tenants listening to their sickening rock music. It was afternoon, and the apartment began to feel warm and close. Lenny dozed for a half hour in his chair, with the dog asleep leaning against his chest. This, I thought, is why I have always loved Lenny. He really is a poet locked up inside a tax-shelter salesman. But now, I thought, he sees the world plain and he will start to live his own life, not Joel's or someone else's, and he will be well. He will reclaim the inner Lenny, who had nothing to do with tax and everything to do with redwood trees and beauty.

But when Lenny awoke from his nap, he got up, drank yet another Diet Pepsi, and then washed his face. "You know what I have to do?" he asked me.

"Move somewhere far away with Linda," I suggested.

"No way," he said. "Those guys from New York were really impressed with my idea. I can find some guys who really like it and won't whine about the tax consequences. Then we'll be off to the races. If I can put this deal together, we'll never have to worry about money again. The pressure'll be off, and Linda and I can really enjoy ourselves. We can start to do the things that we really enjoy."

I shook my head and Lenny said, "What's wrong? Was that Fuchs guy right? Is there a tax problem?"

"Jesus, Lenny," I said. "You made so much sense a few minutes ago. What're you doing now? You're just killing yourself all over again."

"Oh, that," he said. "That was just me feeling sorry for myself. That doesn't get you anywhere in this world. Nobody's giving anything away, are they?" He shrugged his shoulders, and he was Lenny Brown, drug-addicted young American, once again. I drove home, thinking for some reason of Kenneth Fearing and a poem called "McKade." The only line I could remember was, "Sleep, McKade, You are a gentleman and important. Yawn and go to sleep." I cannot remember why I thought of it now.

LOS ANGELES, WINTER 1979-80
THE DEATH OF LENNY BROWN

Lenny Brown never leaves his room by day. He lies in bed on a soiled bed cover, watching "Wedding Day" and munching from a half-empty yellow plastic bowl of Doritos. He lives in Venice now. He is not on the boardwalk, but still there is a gentle breeze which blows across the beach, across the roller skaters on the boardwalk, and finds its way to Lenny Brown's apartment. Lenny does not let it in. The windows are closed. They are covered with soot, in any event. Thick fifth-hand curtains cover the windows. An air conditioner is always running, bringing in the only kind of air that Lenny wants: thoroughly conditioned, strained, filtered air, air that has been frisked on its way into Lenny's apartment to make certain that it is not carrying any concealed weapons.

On the night table next to Lenny's bed there is perpetually a metal ashtray filled to overflowing with half-smoked Viceroys, always smoldering with some vestige of fire, like Mount Saint Helen's, like Lenny. Next to the Viceroys is a Smith and Wesson .38 Python revolver. Lenny likes for people to know he's heeled. In his line of business, a man has to have some respect.

Lenny watches television all day, smokes cigarettes, reads the *Wall Street Journal* and *Forbes*, and then sleeps intermittently. Occasionally he calls about a three-million-dollar property in Bel-Air, makes an appointment but never keeps it. He uses a different name every time. Lately, he has been using Iranian names, like Ammadi and Jahanshah.

For a long time, Lenny made those appointments and kept them. That was when he still thought Linda might be coming back. He would call Coldwell, Banker about the most expensive house in Bel-Air, and then he would drag me along to go see it. The real-estate agents, mostly women who drove Rolls convertibles and looked toughened enough to frighten a lizard, automatically assumed that Lenny was in the record business and that I was his manager. Lenny fostered the illusion by asking me questions such as, "Ben, how much would this really cost me after tax?" and, "Ben, what about using this room as a studio? Could we take an ITC on the whole house?"

Like a computer that has been programmed with a few key phrases so that it can make airline reservations, Lenny still knew quite a few phrases from the days of glory. Computers do not suffer, though, as far as we know, and Lenny was surely suffering plenty. I never knew the point of the trips to Chalon Drive and Funchal Road and Bellagio Terrace. Lenny told me after each house that he thought it was perfect. If he could swing just one deal, he could buy that house, "for cash," always "for cash," and just show it to Linda, and she would know it was time to come back to him. He would talk about the huge living room and the eat-in kitchen and the pool house and cool white sheets in a bedroom the size of an armory and that it had been owned by Johnny Carson's lawyer, and that would be Lenny's plan to get Linda back.

But each trip must have strengthened Lenny's knowledge that he would never get Linda back. First, each time he went to see a mansion in Bel-Air, he knew he would never buy it, could never buy it. Therefore, he could never buy Linda. Second, each time he saw it, he saw how small he was and how large the price of the house was, and that, too, made him ill with self-loathing. Finally, he never encountered any homeowners who had gotten their houses by lying in bed, reading the trades of real estate, dreaming of deals in Bahrain when they dealt 'ludes at night. Somehow, as Lenny once told me in a flash of reality, his line of work does not generally seem to lead to Stone Canyon Road.

All of this meant that Linda was long gone, and indeed she was.

Lenny might have imagined her as the mistress of ceremonies in a house next to the Bel-Air Hotel, but, in fact, she was living a life of utmost quiet in Pacific Palisades. She had moved in with Dr. Tom right after she left the hospital. She had come home one day while Lenny was off on his rounds for Mark. She took a few things and left almost everything of any usefulness in the apartment. She also wrote Lenny a note, which he did not ever let me see, but which I saw one day nevertheless, but that is getting ahead of the story.

Dr. Tom would never be the one love of Linda's life the way she was to him. But Dr. Tom was safe. He did not begin each day with a silent shriek of self-hatred and self-destruction. He did not hate her for simply being around to witness his wrecking of himself. He took care of himself and went through the day. He did not ever take drugs or even drink. He had the idea that if you stayed out of trouble, that was the most fun you could have. He never went to fancy restaurants. He never flew private planes to Acapulco or Las Vegas. He did not gamble or show off. He just wanted to tend his garden at the hospital, come home in the evening, read books about Indian history, and then go to sleep.

He owned a small house on a road in Pacific Palisades. It had only two bedrooms and a small backyard. It had no view of anything except the neighbors' backyards, which was fine with Dr. Tom. "I get my really great views by reading and by thinking," he said, "and if I want to see a great view of the ocean, I can always drive to the beach." The house had only one television set, a standard-issue Sony Trinitron.

Dr. Tom was a practical man. His father had been a gold trader who had been utterly wiped out by a market maneuver against him so complex that I never understood it. The experience had left Dr. Tom with a strong wish to be left alone. He drove a Saab, wore businesslike clothing, and literally walked out of the room when people started to boast about money. I often wonder how he wound up in Los Angeles, but then there are such things as random chance in this world.

Tom had one further passion: to take care of Linda. He was in many ways a womanly man, by which I intend only the highest kind of compliment. He had no interest in playing cards or going to fights or gambling. He had an interest in saving lives at the hospital, maybe someday making a significant contribution in the field of oncology, and in staying out of trouble. But he really wanted to make certain that Linda never suffered again. Of course, that was impossible, but he wanted her never to have to live in constant fear and anxiety again, never have to swim in a sea of self-hate, never have to see a man she loved slowly slicing off pieces of himself and feeding them to a shark.

Linda did not work when she lived with Dr. Tom. She went to ballet for three hours each morning and for an hour and a half each afternoon. She worked for an organization that took care of lost dogs in the Palisades. She worked with Sabrina Schiller in trying to get cleaner air into Los Angeles. She kept busy every minute for the first few weeks. She did not want to think about the life and the love she had left behind. But after the first month, she knew that she was no longer swimming underwater and that she had begun a genuinely new life.

"It doesn't have the highs and the lows," she told me. "That's obvious. But it does have some sense of being an ongoing enterprise that might last for another month or another year or even a lifetime. I never have the feeling that I'm immortal that I used to have when I was with Lenny," she said one day at La Scala, Malibu (my treat). "But I also don't feel as if I'm trying to claw my way out of my own grave. And Tom is so nice, so concerned. If I have a headache, Tom spends all day checking to see if there's a virus around."

For the first few months, Linda did not give Lenny any idea where she was. "It'll just give him another thing to be crazy about," she said. "I don't want him thinking he has to call me up and impress me. No way." (She still used Lenny's phrases.) "It made him completely crazy with guilt to see what had happened between us, and he was also completely crazy with rage about the baby, even though he never let on. So if I'm not there, he just has to deal with the drugs and the real estate, and that might be a lot easier."

I am still amazed at how little Linda understood about Lenny. The absence of the physical presence of a worry did not soothe Lenny any more than a convict will feel soothed if he is sentenced to die and is not in view of the gallows. Lenny still knew every line of every conversation he had ever had with Linda. He still knew what she wore on their first date (a light blue full skirt). Besides, Lenny's anxiety was a variable of one of those social-science laws: His anxiety expanded to fill all the time available for Lenny to think about it.

Still, Linda thought she was doing well for Lenny, and that counts for something. Linda is still alive, and I think Lenny would be grateful to know that.

At this point, as I look back on Lenny and Linda's life together and apart, a question always comes to me: If Linda was able to summon up the strength to run away from Lenny, why didn't she do more for him all along? There he was, falling into pieces, torn apart by Joel and L.A. and the hopes and obsessions that rend the spirit into shredded flesh and blood. There she was, watching, doing almost nothing about it, letting the threshing machine inside and outside Lenny's head cut him into shark bait. Why didn't she do something?

The answer is fear. Linda was always afraid of Lenny. That was part of his attraction for her. He gave the impression when they first met back at Washington Square of being in control of the ship of their destiny. She never doubted it until the very end. She thought he was the captain and she was the mate. He gave the orders, thought the big thoughts, dreamed the big dreams, made the big mistakes. He lifted them up and laid them low. At all times, he was in charge.

Linda was an old-fashioned girl. She was no hustling woman executive, no hot-eyed militant for anything except to be by Lenny's side. When her world began to fall in upon her, she was too scared of Lenny, of the world that had beaten Lenny, to do anything but follow. Whatever her motives were for taking the 'ludes in Santa Cruz, they were deeply buried indeed. At every visible level, she was still just scared, just following orders, until she went to the hospital.

When she left Lenny, that too came from fear. She did not have the strength to stay with him and fight with him to save himself. She was simply too frightened to do it. She did have the strong fear that she was making the apartment at Franklin and LaBrea even more painful for Lenny. She was afraid that she might have really screwed up the evening at Ma Maison, cost Lenny his new beginning with the Saudis' money.

She did what people do when they are afraid. She fled. She was too scared to stay any longer. She had always been too scared to struggle with Lenny against herself. Now she reached the logical terminus of a scared person in a frightening situation: somewhere else.

For a long time, until I saw the note Linda left for Lenny, I blamed her. But not any longer. Even before the note, I was wrong to blame her. After all, who is unafraid?

The afternoon Lenny got home and saw that Linda had moved out, he moved out, too. He took his Panasonic and Daisy and a few clothes and his Dopp kit and moved up to our house for a week until he could find a new place to live.

This time he did not sit in a tan leather chair and mope. This time he read every article and book he could find about how to get rich in real estate. As far as I am concerned, the two exercises are pretty much the same. Both of them are attempts to bind up wounds so deep that they can never be bound up except by love. Certainly, they cannot be bound up by learning how to make money in developing shopping centers in low-income areas. The problem was never really about money, as Lenny should have known, just as hunger is rarely about food.

The problem on this visit from Lenny was that he literally never slept. He was taking at least ten 'ludes each day, and still he never slept. For five days, he did not once sleep. At the end of that five days, he was so beaten down, so utterly defenseless from fatigue, that we were able to persuade him to do something he should have done a year before.

On the morning of the sixth day, my wife and I drove him to a small hospital near Century City which had a program of drug detoxification that was vouched for by all the major names in Hollywood. That should have made us suspicious, but we were stupid, too. I sometimes think that in L.A. it is a constant whirl of the stupid stealing from the stupider.

The hospital had tinted glass windows facing out toward a huge complex of office buildings. It had extremely pretty nurses with long fingernails and punk pink lipstick. The doctor who talked to me and Lenny looked like a sincere man. He reminded me of a doctor on a TV series. He looked as if he would never rest easy until Lenny was a Rotarian. He told me and Lenny that the program was not inexpensive, but that nothing worthwhile ever is, which was another clue we missed. He also told us that the patient had to undergo a certain amount of psychic stress, but that it was nothing compared with what the usual Quaalude addict went through each day.

In a room with a fake Gauguin of a naked woman holding a basket of fruit below two firm breasts, Lenny signed himself in. I signed papers of financial responsibility. That shows I am a fool, but I have never denied it. Then the doctor took Lenny into the bowels of the program. Lenny looked back at me the way a big yellow Labrador might look back as it is led into the heart of a veterinary practice for a purpose so terrible that the dog cannot even start to fathom it. The dog can only look at its master and search for reassurance.

Lenny was allowed no visitors for two weeks, but he was up and around a lot sooner than that. I learned from Lenny what had happened. The first two days went fine. Lenny still had enough methaqualone coursing through his system to keep him going without much withdrawal. Plus, Lenny made friends in the ward with an extremely famous movie director who was in for the same thing Lenny was in for. Lenny and the movie director had several very serious talks about Lenny's organizing a program of movie directors investing their funds in commercial properties. Lenny could offer a way to cut out the enormous general partners' fees that usually totally wrecked such programs. This was a chance for the movie directors to make money with their money and for once be the first people who got a crack at a good property and not the last.

The famous director said that it sounded like a great project to him, but that he wanted to be cut in for a percentage of Lenny's percentage if he were going to introduce Lenny to all those other producers who had money in their pockets.

Then each one would go in for his daily doses of methadone. That was the whole goddam program, for which Lenny and I were paying four hundred dollars each day. Lenny refused to take the methadone after two days. It was making him drowsy all the time. By the third day, he became irritable. At noon, he began to threaten the nurses. By six, he had thrown a Diet Pepsi can against a wall. By nine, he had taken a swing at an orderly. By midnight, he was bleeding profusely from the wrists after cutting at them with the point of a Pentel Fine Line Rolling Writer pen. The famous movie director called the nurses, who brought him to surgery to be patched up.

Lenny had not seen one psychiatrist for even one moment. No one had even talked to him except to show him where his room was and to ask him whether he wanted a kosher plate, the dieter's plate or the ordinary high-protein regimen.

Nevertheless, on the fourth day, while Lenny was still groggy from an immense intravenous dose of Nembutal, they strapped him onto a table covered with light blue leatherette (which made Lenny think of the skirt Linda had worn on their first date), and they gave him "micro-doses" of electroconvulsive therapy each four hours. In response to Lenny's cries for Linda and for the house on Hollywood Boulevard and the Saudi investors and someone to tell him he had done good, the good doctors gave him electroshock so strong that he had to have a polystyrene chock in his mouth so that he did not bite off his tongue.

The shock treatment lasted for six days, night and day. It was like something out of *Darkness at Noon*. By the time it was over, Lenny would have done anything. The shock was supposed to have totally scrambled the receptors in his brain that craved the drug. It was not supposed to make him into a vegetable, but of course it did, temporarily.

When Dr. Silbergeld came to see me in the waiting room on the tenth day, he told me that Lenny had done so well with microdoses of ECS that he could leave the hospital, although the deposit for the full two weeks was not refundable.

When they led Lenny out, he looked like a drugged Frankenstein's monster. At first, he did not recognize me, but then he touched my arm and, in a voice which came from outer space, he said, "You've been a really good friend to me, Benjy. I'll never forget it." He turned the radio to a classical music station, and then he said, "I think I'll be all right now."

In Lenny's eyes, far at the back behind the brown pupils, there was the little wrinkle of terror that appears only in the eyes of people who have been in mental hospitals. The look said that Lenny had stared hell in the eyes, and hell did not blink. That night, we ate at home on our deck overlooking the smoggy San Fernando Valley. Lenny did not talk throughout the meal. Afterward, he smoked a Viceroy and then he said to me, in a tone of utmost gravity and calmness, "Now that I've settled down, I'll be able to concentrate on getting the really important things I want out of life. Without the 'ludes, I can put deals together extremely quickly and bring them to market without any personal resistance."

Lenny sounded like a cross between a computer and a somnambulist (which is perhaps what modern man is). At any rate, the treatment had not worked. That was crystal clear. If Lenny were still obsessed with struggle for a *thing* that would bring salvation, Lenny was destined to be back on 'ludes soon.

Indeed, he was. After a few days of searching, Lenny found a small apartment in Venice, near Navy Street, just a block and a half from the filthy boardwalk. That would be his last move. Of course, Lenny now had absolutely no way to make a living (in his mind) except to deal 'ludes. After all, that was a subject and a skill he knew well by now. The ECS had not made the slightest impression on his life of ambition, self-defeat, and slow suicide. It had speeded up the pace and done no more. ECS cannot shock away a person's entire personality structure of longing and needing unless the doses are so powerful that they make the patient into a permanent vegetable. Lenny had been a vegetable for a few days, but after that he was identical to his pattern.

And yet, to be fair, apparently sometimes the treatment has helped people. It just depends upon what is inside the patient and not on what is outside. The phenomenon reminds me of coyotes. The tan coyote can come near a household dog, look at it, wag its tail, and run away. Yet the brown coyote, *so similarly marked*, will shriek with rage and tear the pet's throat out. There are different levels of pain, of rage, of the need to still the pain.

In Venice, though, Lenny was not going to be a messenger boy for Mark. After an interval when Lenny could not get out of bed, which I have already described, he put deals together and brought them to market without personal resistance. He simply "accessed" Mark's suppliers, told them he would get a dollar more per 'lude, and was in business for himself for the first time in his life. Now, Lenny was dealing in the hundreds and not in dozens. That made the little Python next to the bed a key selling tool. Tough-looking people with woolen ski caps came into Lenny's apartment for thirty seconds at a time. Money changed hands. Lenny tested the 'ludes. He diluted the cash flow by about fifteen percent by his "testing" of the product. He was more or less in a stupor the whole time he was in Venice, but it was a sad, heartbreaking stupor of nightmares of trying to race through mud and swamps, of constantly falling behind, of perpetual danger of humiliation and destruction. Unlike most junkies, Lenny still made schemes of how he would get rich quick in real property. But like many junkies, Lenny narcotized the knowledge of futility with chemicals.

After Lenny had been in Venice for a few months, he got a surprising visitor. Linda defied Dr. Tom's most urgent orders and came to visit Lenny. She had heard of his whereabouts, his business, and his life from me. She knew that he was in terrible condition. In fact, she had gotten the clear impression that he would not have much life expectancy in his current line of work if the typical pattern of Quaalude dealers held good for him, too. And so Linda came to Venice Beach to plead with Lenny to spare himself.

Lenny and Linda had not seen each other since the night at Ma Maison (I still would like to kill the proprietor for what he did to Lenny that night). Linda often asked about Lenny through me. She had a little bit of money saved up from her temporary jobs before she met Dr. Tom. She often asked me to see if Lenny needed food or a visit to a doctor or anything she could buy him with a small amount of money. But Linda did not talk to Lenny on the telephone for reasons I have already discussed. Briefly, she did not want to place him under any further stress, she says.

Was that true? Did Linda still have any feeling for Lenny? You may have gotten the impression that Linda was selfish to abandon Lenny. You might think that I dislike her for having allowed Lenny to be alone, which was what he hated the most. Sometimes I feel that way myself. In the final analysis, Linda probably should have stayed with Lenny. I am convinced that Lenny would be alive now if she had. She simply would not have permitted him to sink as low as he sank without her to give him some feeling of being rooted. But Linda left Lenny out of genuinely understandable motives. She was scared and tired and defeated. She needed to breathe. She had been told by Lenny that he believed she had turned against him. He never seemed to be happy to see her. When she left, she might have really and truly thought she was doing him a favor. She *knew* she was doing herself a favor. And yet, she loved Lenny. I believe she would have cut her own tongue out of her mouth if she thought she could have saved Lenny. She would have turned tricks on Hollywood Boulevard and La Brea if she genuinely thought she could turn Lenny's life around. In fact, it was absolutely clear after Lenny died that Linda loved Lenny as much as one human being can love another. She loved Lenny to an almost frightening degree, almost eerily.

But when he began to hit her, she thought that she had involuntarily become part of the process that was killing her beloved Lenny and not helping her. That was why she left. If this sounds confused, well, life is confusing.

Linda knocked on the door of Lenny's apartment in Venice. Even before she stopped knocking, she knew she was in the right place. It was incredibly filthy, with cats rummaging in garbage at the end of the hall. But it was also home for her Lenny and Daisy. By that kind of brilliant intuition that animals have, Daisy knew it was her mother. She began to bark and throw herself against the door. By the kind of intuition that people who are totally united in love can have, Lenny also knew it was Linda. Normally, he did not answer his door unless he knew specifically the exact moment when someone was arriving. Otherwise, you ended up with a razor across your throat. But this time Lenny knew somehow that it was Linda.

When Lenny answered the door, Linda was actually embarrassed at how healthy she looked. Lenny looked like Lazarus of the beach cities, reeking of stale tobacco smoke, unshaven, hair flying in every direction, mouth open in a kind of dazed grin, brown eyes dull from fatigue and anxiety. He wore grimy black trousers and a black T-shirt. As he registered in his mind that Linda was at the door, he turned to Daisy, who was already leaping up on Linda, and said, "It's your mommy, Daisy."

Linda kissed Lenny on the lips, but just a brush and certainly not the beginning of anything romantic. Lenny offered Linda a chair. He had to sweep several used plastic baggies off its burned green upholstery. Then he offered Linda a Diet Pepsi or a Coke. "I have both," he said. "I cater to every kind of vice."

Linda sat down gingerly in her baggy blue jeans and oxford-cloth shirt. She had the overwhelmingly upsetting feeling that she was visiting the dwelling of *a total stranger*, a college roommate who turned out to be a Hare Krishna chanter. Only in the excitement which he could not really suppress was there the old Lenny. The room, the smell of confined cigarette smoke, the aura of overwhelming mess—the apartment looked just the way she had always imagined Robert Thornton's apartment would look—were the outward signs of a man Linda did not know.

Since I was not there and Linda rarely talks about the event, I can offer only sketchy details of the meeting. Linda told Lenny that she was terribly sorry about leaving him. She felt it was for everyone's good. Lenny said that he had been a total maniac, and it was really amazing that Linda had not left sooner. He said that he missed Linda, but he understood she was living a really good, clean life, and that was important. "It makes me happy to know that someone can still get out of this trap," he said, without specifying which trap as if there were any question.

They talked for a while about Pet Orphans. Incredibly, even in his present style of life, Lenny still sent a contribution to the organization each month. Lenny and Linda swapped stories about pets in distress, about a fox that Linda had seen walking down the street in Pacific Palisades, about how there should be a law against people carrying around dogs loose in the back of pickup trucks, about how it should be a capital offense to abandon a poor little dog that doesn't have any idea of what to do if it isn't with its master.

Lenny giggled to show that he thought that was exactly what Linda had done to him. Then he cleared his throat and said, "No, you didn't abandon me. I ran away. I'm a runaway lost dog."

Linda saw him right then and there as what he was: the dog on the center divider of the freeway. Terrified beyond endurance, absolutely crazed with fear by the rush of traffic and life and speed, driven literally insane so that he needed drugs to survive even when he was taken off the freeway. And yet, she knew, he had been happy sitting in Heinrich's sporting-goods store in Santa Cruz, in the quiet mornings when there was no one around.

As if he could read her mind, he said, "I think about life in Santa Cruz a lot. I wish we were still there. I can remember every meal we ate. I can remember the sound of the ocean on West Cliff Drive."

Linda stared at Lenny and said, "Would you like to go back to Santa Cruz?"

Lenny sat bolt upright and said, "Are you really ready to go? You'd go just like that?"

That was the final turning point of Lenny's life. Linda hesitated for just a moment, and that was long enough for Lenny to slouch back in his chair and say, "Oh, you meant by myself. Of course. That was really stupid of me. Really, really stupid. I thought you meant both of us."

For a wild moment, like a Russian prince hazarding his entire estate on the turn of a card, Linda hesitated again and thought maybe she would. Maybe she was meant to be on this roller coaster forever, to have the wild highs and the lows. Maybe that was what life was about and not about being like a certificate of deposit in a safe-deposit box, paying a little bit of interest every quarter, sleeping the rest of the time.

But Lenny picked up on the hesitation and not on the thought and said, "That would be crazy of you. You have such a good thing going for you right now."

And yet, and yet. Linda could start to feel the blood rising in her again. She could feel the way she felt when Lenny held her in the swimming pool, the way she felt the first time he took her for a drink after poetry class at NYU, the overwhelming feeling, like a tide crashing on a beach, that she was with the only man she would ever totally love.

Lenny said, "Never mind. I'm not going anywhere. I'm getting almost enough of a stake together to buy a little office building. Right here in Venice. Then I can demolish it and put in a high-rise condo project. I have the investors lined up. You meet a lot of rich people dealing real 'ludes, not boots." He said that and he lit up a cigarette, and Linda knew that she would go back to Dr. Tom that afternoon and stay.

Linda said, "I want you to go into a treatment program, Lenny." She stroked Daisy's hair and said, "I think there are places that can help you. Not like that horror show in Century City. I think there are real places. Maybe the Menninger place in Kansas."

Lenny said, "I don't need any *places*. I don't need any places for crazy people. If you think I'm crazy"—and then he paused and laughed— 'I don't blame you, but I'm not. Crazy people do not make seven hundred dollars a week tax free."

Linda said, "There are plenty of crazy people in L.A. making a million dollars a month tax free."

"You've got me there," Lenny said. "But I'm not crazy. I took a few wrong turns. I made a lot of mistakes. Plus, I'm not gonna lie to you. It's real hard to concentrate as well as I should because I miss having you around. I keep turning to say things to you, and you're not there. I've been turning around to tell you how pretty you look for about four months now, and you're never there. I remember how pretty you looked that night at Ma Maison. God, you made all those movie stars look sick. I keep turning around to tell you that, but you're not there, and then it takes me a while to concentrate again."

Linda began to cry at that point. Through her tears, she grasped Lenny's hand and said, "Lenny, please go somewhere and get help. Please. Please. I'll pay for it. I'll work two jobs. I'll do anything. Please get straightened out. I know there are places."

Lenny hugged Linda while the dog, Daisy, licked at Linda's tears.

"I don't need any *places*," Lenny said. "It makes me feel really good to know you're concerned, and that's a lot better than any places. Plus, if I can just put together a really nice score in Venice while real estate here is still going up by leaps and bounds, I'll be all set. You'll see. In five years, we'll be laughing about all this as if it happened to someone else."

As if it happened to someone else. But it wasn't happening to someone else. It was happening to Lenny Brown, the man whom Linda loved more than she loved anything else in the world, and if you ask her why she didn't stay with Lenny that night if she loved him more than anything else, she will only cry and shake her head, and you will have been a fool for having asked why men and women in love do what they do.

Linda left. Lenny walked her out to her Volvo station wagon, squinting in the sun. He had not been out in daylight for a long time. He hugged her and brushed her on the lips. "I'm going to get you some new clothes," she said. "I remember your size."

Good-bye, they said. Lenny said he had better get back into the house because he was expecting his biggest shipment of 'ludes ever, over a thousand real ones, and he did not want to miss the appointment which was in only a few minutes. He looked up and down Pacific Street to see if there were any likely DEA cars, and then he hugged Linda again and said, "It'll be all right, It'll all be all right in the end."

Then he squeezed her hand three times. *I love you.* She squeezed back *I love you too.* Then she thought she would break down, so she left.

Linda drove north on Pacific to Main Street, Santa Monica, and then up the Pacific Coast Highway, where she had tried to take Lenny for a picnic. When she got back to the neat clean house in the Palisades, she remembered that she had not asked how Daisy was getting along. She called Lenny, but no one answered.

She sat in her backyard and cried for a long time. Then she came into the house to make herb-baked chicken, a low-cholesterol dish that was one of Tom's favorites. Even Nathan Pritikin recommended it.

Back in Venice, Lenny called me up. I came over and arrived right after the thousand 'ludes. Lenny showed them to me in ten large plastic bags. "Figure five bucks' profit on each one, and I'm golden. But I'm going to wholesale them out," he said. "A guy is coming to buy them all for a buck-fifty above my cost to take them back to New York. Christ, in New York everybody is taking them now."

Lenny told me about Linda's visit. His voice broke several times, but he was obviously happy that Linda had come to see him. He had cleaned up his apartment and even thrown out all the piles of dead cigarettes. He was working on Windexing a window when I saw him. He actually had the curtains open, and we could smell the ocean over the Windex.

As I write this, I see that maybe it was not Linda's fault for not saying she would go to Santa Cruz with him. Maybe just her visit had turned the tide, and Lenny would have gotten back to dry land with her just coming over to teach him how to walk again. But probably not. Lenny would have cleaned up the apartment and then gotten discouraged about something in a real-estate agent's office and then come home and stewed in smoldering Viceroys for another month, plotting his comeback.

Lenny and I went out for a drink at the West Beach Cafe. It was deserted. The white walls and modern art under brilliant lights were stark and depressing. Lenny talked about how, if he could do a few deals like this every month, he would soon be sitting pretty. He ate spinach rigatoni, drank several glasses of red wine, and then we walked home.

I left him at the entrance to his apartment house. There were only about twenty feet between me and my car when I left him, but I still felt nervous. Venice was, and is, a place of violence. Lenny said he would call me when he had gotten his seventy-five hundred bucks, and maybe if I were still up typing, he would take me and my wife for a late drink at the Polo Lounge. By now it was after dark, and Lenny was in an almost festive mood. Amazingly, he said something extremely similar to me to what he had told Linda. "This is the turning point," he said. "In a year, in six months, we won't believe that I was living like this. *It'll be like it happened to someone else.*"

Perhaps that is how all people who suffer cope with the pain. They imagine that it is happening to someone else, or that someday they will think it happened to someone else. There are worse ways to deal with suffering and Lenny used them, too.

As I turned to wave good-bye to Lenny, I noticed that there were two huge trucks unloading lights at the end of the block of Lenny's street. The lights were apparently for illuminating a nighttime scene of a movie or TV show. I could see carnival scenery being set up, a small arcade and a horse from a merry-go-round. I made a note to ask Lenny what show it was. Maybe they would want to hire me to write a script. Then I got into my car and waved at Lenny again. He smiled broadly, just as he had when he left me ostensibly to take a taxi, but really to take a subway, back on Cortlandt Street in New York City, long ago, when the whole thing must have seemed to Lenny to be happening to someone else and not the person in a small apartment on Navy Street in Venice, where he had to carry a gun to show he meant business. I could hear Daisy bark as he started up the stairs.

At about midnight, I decided that I would not hear from Lenny about a drink. I put on the radio, the Elvis hour, and heard the KRLA news. The announcer said that there had been a drug-related shooting in Venice and that the police said that a man had been shot fatally in what was thought to be a Quaalude-related theft. Ironically, the announcer added, the street was being used as a backdrop for an episode of "CHiPs" at the very moment the crime occurred.

I arrived in Venice in twenty minutes. I ran every red light and hit 110 on the Santa Monica Freeway. Of course, it was Lenny. He had been hit twice by .38 slugs from his own gun. Once in the neck, once in the chest. There was blood everywhere. Daisy stood next to Lenny's body, quivering and crying. When the police coroner poked at Lenny's chest, Daisy growled at him. I took her in my arms, which she let me do because I knew her. "It's all right," I said to her. "It's all right."

Lenny actually looked as if he were not sad to be dead. His eyes looked surprised, but almost pleasantly surprised. As soon as I saw his face, I thought of the John F. Kennedy line about how the survivors of a nuclear war might envy the dead. Lenny's war was over anyway.

The room had only five live people in it besides me. All of them were from the police. One of the policemen had a gray toupee. He looked at me with watery hazel eyes and told me that it looked as if Lenny had been killed in the middle of a drug buy that went down wrong. The police surmised that because there was a bag with ten 'ludes in it found in the hallway just outside Lenny's apartment door. No one in the building had seen or heard anything suspicious.

The policeman asked me if I knew the victim or was just there as a reporter.

"Both," I said.

I rode down to the morgue with Lenny's body in the back of an ambulance. I did not want him to be alone in his final ride through the city that had mystified and awed and overwhelmed him. We traveled along the Santa Monica Freeway toward downtown and all along the freeway, we could see the lights of Los Angeles, a city which Lenny had loved, and which could not possibly have cared less.

I went east to the funeral. Linda came too, but she flew to Boston first, so we did not see each other except at the service. It was at an old miserable synagogue on a decrepit street near Borough Park. The rabbi obviously had no idea who Lenny was, which, of course, did not make his relationship to Lenny any different from anyone else's. Most of the service was in Hebrew, so it did at least become clear that Lenny had been Jewish, and not Italian or some other ethnic group's progeny. His mother and father looked so bereft that I could not bear to talk to them about why the father had never spoken to him when he was a child, or why the mother had tried to shame a sensitive child and bully him into becoming a colorless grind, or an insensate hustler. When the service was over, I had my driver take Linda straight to the airport for her return to L.A.

"Although, really," she said, "I don't know why I'm going back there. Really, at this point, I don't know why I'm anywhere." She took a round brown Mellaril with water in the car on the way to JFK, and she had actually fallen asleep by the time we reached the terminal. Dr. Tom had prescribed it for her.

I had the driver take me back to the cemetery near Borough Park. It was small and crowded. Most of the Stars of David and stones were from before World War II. The last names had not yet been Americanized. They were foreign, strange-sounding names which rang of ghettos and shrieking for air at Ellis Island and clawing their way out of nowhere to somewhere, a place where you could buy ten shirts at a clip or have your own plane fly you to Vegas to bet eight thousand dollars on one card. In those people's sad, driven lives, I thought, there was just no room for someone who had the sensitivity to pick up a lost dog even if he were late for an important business meeting. There was no room for a man who would give a valet an extra dollar on the day he went bust because the valet looked sad. Of course, there was no room for a man who could be so inspired by the sight of a city's skyline that he thought he would live forever. But that was where Lenny lay, with those people.

Someday, if his parents will let me do it, I would like to have his remains moved to a hillside in Santa Cruz, overlooking the endless green ocean, overhung by a limitless, perfectly azure sky.

A final note. By the time I had gotten back to the apartment on Navy Street, it had been pretty much picked clean. The faithful Panasonic, which Lenny loved the way a mother loves a child, was gone. So was Lenny's radio and even most of his clothes. I had the dog, Daisy, whom I later gave to the children of a very successful television producer, for Linda had not wanted her. It made her too sad to look at her. I visit Daisy sometimes. She always looks sad. She had never wanted anything except Lenny's presence, and now it was gone.

But in a drawer of Lenny's night table was a packet of letters. Most of them were almost ten years old. They had apparently been written by Linda to Lenny when they first met, even though they saw each other every day in Modern American Poetry class. Many of the letters were poems themselves. Linda had that side of herself which I had not even known about. But Lenny and Linda were poets. Some of the poems were really superbly written, shaming the efforts of those of us who get paid for writing. I returned those letters to Linda. But I kept one which was dated only a few months before, which was the letter Linda had left for Lenny on the day she moved out of the apartment on La Brea and Franklin and left Lenny spinning like a doomed, lone atom in an unconcerned universe (although both she and I cared, Lenny, and you know it).

Here is the letter she wrote:

Dearest Lenny,

I could always live without your loving me if only you would let me love you. That is the only thing I have ever wanted to do since the first time we met, to love you, to take care of you, to feel as if you were part of me. But I am not so selfish that I will do it even if it makes you crazy to have me around. I am going for a while, maybe forever, but I will always be in touch, through Ben or directly. Please keep this and read it occasionally and know that not a minute goes by that I do not think of you. Here is a little farewell sonata for you to sing yourself to sleep with (remember how you used to love for me to sing you lullabies?).

And here is Linda's farewell sonata to Lenny:

Is there still any sign there, any shadow or mark,
On the concrete paths of Washington Square in the rain,
Where we talked about how beauty would change the
    world
And laughed and kissed and stood still?

Is there noise of secrets and cries and sighs
Along the snowy paths of Central Park where we huddled
Together against the cold and knew that we alone could
Keep us alone warmer than fire,
Is there any sound at all?

Is there any footstep in the paths of Santa Cruz,
In the redwood forests so thick we could hide in them
   forever
And never have to come out to see the harsh sun,
And broken trail of breadcrumbs so that we could find our
   way
Back to home, that perfect word, any sign at all?

There must be signs, tokens of all these things,
For those were soaring hours, the diamond moments
Of life for two whole human beings and if there are no
   signs
Of our passage, then life would be too hard
And not at all the emerald of beauty we talked of in
Washington Square Park.

There must be a shadow of our hour in places
Where we talked and felt and knew, yes, knew
That the world of light and sun was a gorgeous place.
But if there is no shadow of our hopes left in the
World of light, then there must be a shadow for us
In darkness, and when you find it, I will meet you there
Forever.

That is Linda's farewell sonata. Goddam you, Lenny, come back.

DATE LOANED

MAR 1 6 1984			

HIGHSMITH 45-222

GARDNER-WEBB COLLEGE LIBRARY
P. O. Box 836
Boiling Springs, N.C. 28017

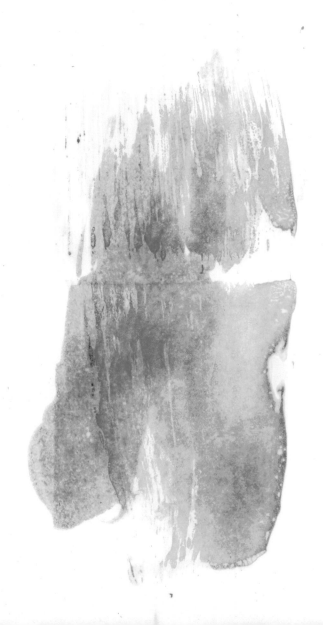